UNDERSTANDING REPRODUCTIVE LOSS

Understanding Reproductive Loss
Perspectives on Life, Death and Fertility

Edited by

SARAH EARLE
The Open University, UK

CAROL KOMAROMY
The Open University, UK

LINDA LAYNE
Rensselaer Polytechnic Institute, USA

ASHGATE

Published by
Ashgate Publishing Limited
Wey Court East
Union Road
Farnham
Surrey, GU9 7PT
England

Ashgate Publishing Company
110 Cherry Street
Suite 3-1
Burlington, VT 05401-3818
USA

www.ashgate.com

British Library Cataloguing in Publication Data
Understanding reproductive loss : perspectives on life, death and fertility.
1. Fetal death. 2. Fetal death--Psychological aspects.
3. Infertility, Female. 4. Infertility, Female--
Psychological aspects.
I. Earle, Sarah, 1972- II. Komaromy, Carol, 1948-
III. Layne, Linda L.
362.1'98178-dc23

Library of Congress Cataloging-in-Publication Data
Earle, Sarah, 1972-
Understanding reproductive loss : perspectives on life, death and fertility / by Sarah Earle, Carol Komaromy and Linda Layne.
p. cm.
Includes bibliographical references and index.
ISBN 978-1-4094-2810-7 (hardback) -- ISBN 978-1-4094-2811-4 (ebook) 1. Fetal death--Psychological aspects. 2. Infertility, Female--Psychological aspects. I. Komaromy, Carol, 1948- II. Layne, Linda L. III. Title.

RG631.E27 2012
618.3'92--dc23

2012022130

ISBN 9781409428107 (hbk)
ISBN 9781409428114 (ebk – pdf)
ISBN 9781409472414 (ebk – ePUB)

FSC
www.fsc.org
MIX
Paper from responsible sources
FSC® C018575

Printed and bound in Great Britain by the MPG Books Group, UK.

Contents

List of Figures and Tables

Notes on Contributors

Dorothy Atkinson is Emeritus Professor of Learning Disability in the Faculty of Health and Social Care at the Open University. She was co-founder (with Jan Walmsley) of the university's Social History of Learning Disability research group which has pioneered the use of personal testimony in tracing the 'hidden history' of learning disability.

Zsuzsa Berend teaches sociology at the University of California Los Angeles (UCLA), USA. She has worked on cultural conceptualisations of love, work, and money among nineteenth-century women. More recently, she has been exploring various facets of surrogacy as experienced and articulated by surrogates.

Jan Bleyen currently teaches oral history and anthropological history at the University of Louvain in Belgium. His main interests lay in the history of the body, the senses and emotion, in particular issues dealing with loss. He primarily works on changing mourning culture and the methodology of oral history. In 2005 he published *De dood in Vlaanderen. Opvattingen en praktijken in Vlaanderen na 1950* (*Death in Flanders. Beliefs and Practices since 1950*) with Davidsfonds. He has also published several articles on the history of death, including three chapters in the *Encyclopaedia of Death and the Human Experience* (Sage, 2009). His PhD, *Stillborn: A history of meaning-making*, focused on performativity and is published by De Bezige Bij, Amsterdam: Doodgeboren.

Ruth Cain is Lecturer in Law at the University of Kent, UK. She is interested in the study of law, gender and reproductive issues from interdisciplinary perspectives. She has recently published in *Feminist Legal Studies* (vol 17, August 2009) on legal and cultural interpretations of maternal depression, and is working on a book project on the disciplining and regulation of modern mothers through law, media and popular discourse, to be published by Zed Books.

Anna Davidsson Bremborg is a parish minister in the Church of Sweden and is affiliated to the University of Lund, Sweden. Her major research field is thanatosociology with studies of funeral directors, representations of dead bodies and memorialisation of stillborn. Among her publications are her thesis *Occupation: Funeral Director* (2002, in Swedish) and the chapter 'Dead Bodies on the Internet' in *Making Sense of Death, Dying and Bereavement: An Anthology*, ed. by S. Earle, C. Bartholomew and C. Komaromy (Sage, 2009).

Karen Dyer is a PhD candidate in medical anthropology at the University of South Florida. Her research focuses on reproductive decision-making and infertility among cancer survivors in Puerto Rico as an integral aspect of long-term cancer survivorship. Using a critical-interpretive approach, Dyer examines how the experience of infertility and the desire for parenthood change in the context of life-threatening disease.

Sarah Earle is Senior Lecturer and Associate Dean for Research in the Faculty of Health & Social Care at The Open University, UK. She is interested in reproductive and sexual health and has published widely in these areas. Her co-edited publications include *Gender Identity and Reproduction* (Palgrave, 2003); *Sociology for Nurses* (Polity, 2005); *The Sociology of Healthcare* (Palgrave, 2008); *Death and Dying: A Reader* (Sage, 2009); and, *Making Sense of Death, Dying and Bereavement: An Anthology* (Sage, 2009). She is presently sub-editor for the journal *Human Fertility*.

Nicholas Embleton is a consultant neonatal paediatrician, having trained in paediatrics in Newcastle upon Tyne, UK and Vancouver, Canada. He has worked in neonatal medicine for the past 15 years and has a varied research programme.

Allison Farnworth is Senior Research Midwife at Newcastle University, UK. Her general interests are around reproductive care, and the ways in which research evidence is used by organisations and health care practitioners.

Ruth Graham is Senior Lecturer in Sociology in the School of Geography, Politics and Sociology at Newcastle University, UK. She has a general interest in social science perspectives on health and health care. Her most recent work has focused on exploring experiences of receiving and providing health care in relation to reproductive losses, such as termination of pregnancy and neonatal death. This work on reproductive loss forms part of broader research interests that centre on exploring how distressing life events are experienced and how suffering is conceptualised and responded to in social context.

Carol Komaromy is a medical sociologist who has worked as an academic at the Open University since 1994 and has been involved in research and teaching in the area of death and dying. She chairs the highly successful Open University module on death and dying and has been involved in several research projects in end-of-life care. Carol has a practice background in healthcare, midwifery and counselling and is committed to the belief that sociological research should make a difference to the experience of service users and providers. She is co-editor of the journal *Mortality*.

Linda L. Layne is Hale Professor of Humanities and Social Sciences, and Professor of Anthropology at Rensselaer Polytechnic Institute. She has worked on pregnancy loss since 1986 when she had the first of seven miscarriages. In *Motherhood Lost: A Feminist Account of Pregnancy loss in America*, she uses the lens of anthropology to explain why American women are so ill-prepared for miscarriage, stillbirth, or early infant death and why the feminist movement has not fully embraced this important women's health issue. She developed a women's health approach to childbearing loss in an award-winning television series, 'Motherhood Lost: Conversations'. She is editor or co-editor of two books on motherhood and consumption and a collection on *Feminist Technology*. She is currently studying single mothers by choice, two mom, and two dad families.

Gayle Letherby is Professor of Sociology at the University of Plymouth, UK. Research and writing interests include method, methodology and epistemology; reproductive and non/parental identity and gender and health. Recent relevant publications include *Extending Social Research: Application, Implementation and Publication*, with Letherby, G. and Bywaters, P. (2007) (Buckingham: Open University) and *Introduction to Gender: Social Science Perspectives*, with Marchbank, J. and Letherby, G. (2007) (Harlow: Pearson).

Cathy E. Lloyd is Senior Lecturer in the Faculty of Health and Social Care at The Open University, UK. In 1991, after gaining her PhD in Community Medicine (Public Health) at the University of London, she moved to the United States where she coordinated a longitudinal study on the natural history of type 1 diabetes. She then gained an R.D. Lawrence Fellowship from Diabetes UK and went on to study the impact of stress on diabetes. With more than 70 publications to her credit, Cathy has written and taught extensively on psychological factors and diabetes. She is currently Associate Editor of the journal *Diabetic Medicine*.

Kathy Mason is a visiting research associate in the School of Geography, Politics and Sociology, Newcastle University.

Khadija Mitu is a PhD student in the Department of Science and Technology Studies at Rensselaer Polytechnic Institute. Her research focuses on the experiences of cancer patients in the United States facing and dealing with the fertility damaging effects of cancer treatments. Bringing the medical anthropological approach to the science and technology studies, Mitu aims to conduct ethnographic research to critically analyze how the medical practices of oncology and reproductive endocrinology, the policies related to fertility preservation, and support groups affect the experiences of cancer patients and survivors dealing with the adverse effects of cancer treatments on their reproductive health and family life.

Samantha Murphy is Lecturer in Health and Social Care at the Open University, UK. Her PhD thesis which was undertaken at the University of Surrey considered gendered differences in the experience of stillbirth.

Elizabeth Peel is Senior Lecturer in Psychology at Aston University, Birmingham, UK and a Mid-Career Fellow of The British Academy. She is a critical psychologist with research interests in health, sexualities and gender. Her latest book is *Lesbian, Gay, Bisexual, Trans & Queer Psychology: An introduction* (Cambridge University Press, 2010) with Clarke, Ellis and Riggs.

Judith Rankin is Professor of Maternal and Perinatal Epidemiology in the Institute of Health & Society at Newcastle University, UK. Her research programme centres around understanding the aetiology of congenital anomalies in particular how factors such as obesity, diabetes, alcohol, drugs and environmental influences, and assisted technologies affect their occurrence. She also has a research interest in reproductive loss on parents and health professionals. Prof. Rankin is a member of the British Isles Network of Congenital Anomaly Registers (BINOCAR) and is Register lead for the European Surveillance of Congenital Anomaly Registers (EUROCAT).

Stephen Robson (MB BS MRCOG MD) is Professor of Fetal Medicine and a member of the Institute of Cellular Medicine at Newcastle University, UK). His main research interests are; uterine cell signalling, mechanisms of myometrial quiescence and clinical trials in the area of high risk pregnancy and prenatal screening. He has been involved in the development and audit of national guidelines relating to obstetric care and is closely involved with the UK Comprehensive Research Network.

Julie Savage is Lecturer in Sociology and Medical Sociology at North Hertfordshire College, UK. She is currently Course Co-ordinator for the Access to Higher Education Programme. She was responsible for reconstructing the programme which included the development of a new Health and Science Professions Diploma for learners wishing to pursue health-related academic and professional pathways. Her PhD, which was completed part-time through the Open University, focused on women's experiences of pre-eclampsia. Julie has a PGCE and is a Member of the Institute for Learning.

Susannah Thompson was awarded her PhD with Distinction from the School of Humanities at the University of Western Australia in 2008; her thesis focused on the changing attitudes towards peri-natal death in Australia in the twentieth century with a particular focus on women's own responses to the loss of a baby or pregnancy. She has published widely on this topic in a diverse range of scholarly journals and community-based publications. For several years Susannah was Honorary Fellow at the University of Western Australia where she was involved in interdisciplinary teaching with the Department of Anatomy and Human Biology and the School of Humanities. She has also published a social history of an inner-city suburb in Perth, Western Australia.

Liz Tilley is a lecturer in the Faculty of Health and Social Care at the Open University. She completed her PhD in 2006 on advocacy for people with learning disabilities and continues to be involved in researching issues in learning disability policy and practice, drawing on historical perspectives. She is the current chair of the Social History of Learning Disability research group and Convenor of the International Network on the History of Sterilization for Women with Intellectual Disabilities.

Erica van der Sijpt is a medical anthropologist at the University of Amsterdam in the Netherlands. Her PhD research, *Ambiguous Ambitions: On Pathways, Projects, and Pregnancy Interruptions in Cameroon,* which was completed at the Amsterdam Institute for Social Science Research (AISSR), focuses on women's experiences, ideas and practices with regard to pregnancy loss in the East province of Cameroon. Erica's research interests cover issues related to reproductive health, medical practices, body politics, gender, kinship, religion, and demography.

Cecilia Vindrola-Padros recently obtained her PhD in medical anthropology from the University of South Florida, USA. Her doctoral research took place in Argentina and focused on the experiences of paediatric oncology patients who had to travel to the capital of Buenos Aires in order to access medical treatment. Her areas of interest for research include: child health/hospitalisation, medical migration/travel/tourism, parenting, health policy, cancer treatment, oncofertility, critical medical anthropology, and narrative research. She is currently a research consultant at the Center of Excellence for Aging and Brain Repair.

Jan Walmsley is Visiting Chair in the History of Learning Disabilities at the Open University and an independent consultant/researcher. Her interest in gender and learning disability dates from her PhD, *Gender, Caring and Learning Disability* (1995) and she has subsequently researched and published on this topic. She is co-author of *Towards a Good Life for People with Intellectual Disabilities* (Policy Press 2010).

Kate Woodthorpe is Lecturer in Sociology at the University of Bath, UK. Her research interests centre on the disposal of bodies, the presentation/interpretation of grief through memorialisation, and the professionalisation of bereavement services.

An Introduction to Understanding Reproductive Loss

Sarah Earle, Carol Komaromy and Linda Layne

In 2007 the Open University hosted a symposium jointly organised by the British Sociological Association's Human Reproduction Study Group and the University's Birth and Death Research Group, funded by a grant from the Foundation for the Sociology of Health and Illness. The symposium, *Making a difference: Experiences of reproduction and loss*, brought together key stakeholders in the arena of reproductive loss including policy-makers, practitioners, researchers, academics and service users to provide a timely opportunity for those involved in working and researching within this field to share their knowledge with one another, and to learn from, and share their knowledge with, those who have themselves experienced loss. Following the success of this symposium, a conference focusing on *Experiencing reproductive loss: Working together to change practice* was held in 2008 at the Open University. This conference, and symposium, brought together a growing number of people interested in understanding reproductive loss, and their commitment and enthusiasm led to the development of this book.

Rethinking Reproductive Loss

Reproductive loss is experienced in diverse ways and we use this term to highlight this diversity and to show the fluidity of definitions, understandings and experiences. The study of human reproduction has often focused on reproductive 'success' or – at the very least – on the struggle to achieve reproductive success, rather than on reproductive 'failures', or experiences of loss (Earle et al. 2008). Social scientists have noted that the discourses which surround pregnancy and childbirth focus on positive outcomes and 'happy endings' without acknowledging that reproductive loss is a common and frequently repeated experience. Layne (2003: 1881), for example, argues that: '… emphasis on happy endings, whether believed to be the result of medical intervention or women's natural inborn powers to reproduce, exacerbates the experience of those whose pregnancies do not end happily'. Here, we use the term 'reproductive loss' not only to refer to experiences of early and late miscarriage, termination of pregnancy, stillbirth, perinatal and infant death, as well as maternal death – but also to other kinds of losses relating to reproduction including the loss of 'normal' reproductive experience such as that associated with infertility, assisted reproduction and the medicalisation of pregnancies, labours and deliveries defined as 'high risk'. We also use this term to address all experiences of non-normative reproduction to include the curtailment of reproductive futures and desires, whether by individual action or social structures.

In this book we seek to offer an approach that is non-hierarchical in that it does not try, or want, to categorise experiences of loss in a way that some might be seen as more 'serious' or more 'traumatic' than others. Given the variety of experiences that might be brought under the broad umbrella of reproductive loss it seems reasonable to imagine that there would also be a wide range of responses. Whilst many people will experience loss as intensely devastating, some of the chapters in this book show that other responses are also possible in that reproductive loss can result in ambivalence, or feelings that are not easily expressed.

Experiences of reproductive loss vary. However, there are also some commonalities and this book explores issues of difference and diversity, as well as sameness. In doing so it offers a range of multidisciplinary perspectives and draws on a variety of empirical, theoretical and methodological approaches.

An Overview of Chapters

The first five chapters in the book focus on the loss of normative reproductive expectations. They also consider the loss of anticipated, reproductive futures and desires and the implications of this for people's lives, and for policy and practice.

Chapter 1, by Gayle Letherby, draws on sociological auto/biography – which locates the individual within the social, and highlights the relationship between the self and others – to explore 'infertility' and 'involuntary childlessness'. Following a miscarriage over twenty-five years ago, and drawing on her own experiences of infertility, involuntary childlessness and non-motherhood, Letherby explains how the losses she experienced are often misunderstood and under-researched. In particular, she notes how the status and experiences associated with the identities of defining oneself, or being defined as infertile and/or childless, are complex and varied, as are their related losses, ambivalences and resolutions.

Chapter 2, written by Liz Tilley, Jan Walmsley, Sarah Earle and Dorothy Atkinson offers an international perspective on the involuntary sterilisation of women with intellectual disabilities, drawing predominantly on evidence from modern Western societies, with a particular emphasis on the UK. Using oral history, life story approaches, social policy and health sociology, Tilley, Walmsley, Earle and Atkinson explore a long history of the sterilisation of women with intellectual disabilities which was fairly widespread until the 1970s. In this chapter they argue that it would be a mistake to consider this practice a historical aberration, since similar practices – including social and chemical sterilisation – continue today to constrain the reproductive futures of women with intellectual disabilities. However, just as Letherby highlights the ambivalences that are associated with infertility, involuntarily childlessness and non-motherhood, Tilley, Walmsley, Earle and Atkinson note that sterilisation practices might also produce ambivalence and create opportunities and freedoms, as well as experiences of loss.

In Chapter 3, Karen Dyer, Khadija Mitu and Cecilia Vindrola-Padros adopt a comparative approach to consider the social shaping of fertility loss following treatment for cancer. Locating their work within the interdisciplinary field of oncofertility – which addresses both the biological and sociocultural aspects of iatrogenic infertility with a view to developing policies aimed at the promotion of fertility preservation – the authors note that since more people are surviving cancer (particularly so in developed countries), healthcare providers are increasing their attention to longer-term quality of life issues, including the adverse secondary health effects of treatment on reproductive choices and futures. In this chapter, which focuses on oncofertility in the US, Puerto Rico and Argentina, Dyer, Mitu and Vindrola-Padros argue that access to treatment and reproductive technologies are shaped by a number of factors including the ideologies that underpin the organisation of health systems, government health policies, biomedical practices, as well as individual action. Understanding how these diverse factors influence patient experience, they argue, can inform policies designed to reduce inequalities.

The fourth chapter considers the experience of pre-eclampsia – one of the most common complications in pregnancy. Julie Savage draws on an in-depth qualitative study conducted in the UK to show how reproductive expectations are reconstructed after suffering from this potentially life-threatening condition. In this Chapter, Savage argues that women begin their reproductive journeys by assuming that pregnancy and childbirth are 'natural' and 'normal', thus marginalising any perceived risks. As the symptoms of pre-eclampsia emerge, women re-evaluate their experiences of pregnancy and come to see it as inherently risky, developing varying strategies to manage this risk. Savage concludes by arguing that health practitioners should better understand women's expectations of pregnancy and childbirth, since this can providc insight into how women might respond within the context of emerging problematic symptoms. Moreover, she argues that if the role of the midwife is to be 'with women' then they should fully engage with pregnancies defined as 'abnormal', as well as those seen as 'normal', to ensure that all women can receive woman-centred care that is informative, supportive and even empowering.

Continuing with the theme of complications in pregnancy, Chapter 5, written by Sarah Earle and Cathy Lloyd, examines the experience of diabetes in pregnancy, arguing that this experience sits at the very centre of a paradox in which anticipated normalcy is juxtaposed against a disease experience. By drawing on the social sciences literature in this area, and on the findings of a research consultation process involving women with pre-existing and gestational diabetes in the UK, the authors explore how women with diabetes experience a series of reproductive losses throughout the pregnancy process. However, Earle and Lloyd argue that loss is not just experienced during pregnancy, childbirth and early motherhood but, for some women, the experience of diabetes in pregnancy can also influence women's future reproductive decision-making.

In the next five chapters, the different meanings of loss and the way that loss is understood and expressed in different contexts is considered.

Chapter 6 offers a critical feminist analysis of sonographically-diagnosed miscarriage, drawing on lesbian and heterosexual experiential accounts to interrogate the academic and lay literatures surrounding pregnancy loss. In this Chapter, Elizabeth Peel and Ruth Cain argue that heteronormativity marginalises the experiences of lesbians – and other women located outside of the heterosexual 'norm' – and that engagement with such non-normative experiences can enhance understandings of miscarriage and contribute to feminist social sciences. The authors conclude that pregnancy loss literature should make women aware of the possibility that ultrasound can reveal pregnancy loss, and that health professionals should ensure women receive timely information following such an experience that takes into account their relational situation.

In Chapter 7, Zsuzsa Berend uses cyber-ethnography to analyse discussions of pregnancy loss on one of the largest support websites for surrogate mothers in the US: www.surromomonline.com. Whilst the author argues that surrogacy offers other women the possibility to fulfil their dreams and desires of becoming a mother, surrogate pregnancy loss can be experienced as painfully traumatic, even though surrogates disclaim any attachment to the foetus(s) they carry. Although surrogates are especially vulnerable to feelings of failure when a pregnancy fails, this cyber-ethnography demonstrates they are denied sympathy at the loss even more so than women who are pregnant with their own child. In this Chapter Berend argues that whilst all forms of pregnancy loss are taboo, this is felt particularly keenly by surrogates who can sometimes undergo extreme physical and emotional trauma in their pursuit to give others 'the gift of life'.

Chapter 8, written by Erica van der Sijpt, draws on 15 months of anthropological fieldwork in a village in the East Province of Cameroon in Western Central Africa. The chapter explores how women of the local Gbigbil community think and talk about different forms of reproductive loss and how these ideas connect with the biomedical time-based distinction that frames conventional understandings of loss in Western contexts. Here, van der Sijpt argues that – with some exceptions – in Western societies there is often a persistent effort to demarcate between different types of reproductive loss and that these demarcations are made on the basis of fixed temporal divisions. In contrast, the author shows that in non-Western contexts, different forms of pregnancy loss are distinguished on the basis of other criteria that have little to do with foetal or maternal age, or any other temporal classification. Exploring the Gbigbil concepts of 'force' and 'form', van der Sjipt argues that in this part of eastern Cameroon, reproductive events can, in fact, define the relevance of biomedical time-based models of reproductive loss, rather than be defined and determined by them.

Samantha Murphy considers the way in which parents struggle with constructions of parenthood following the birth of a stillborn baby in Chapter 9. Using symbolic interactionism, Murphy draws on a sociological study of couples bereaved by stillbirth, some of whom were interviewed together as a couple and others individually. She argues that the term 'bereaved parent' is actually a contradiction in terms since people bereaved by stillbirth might experience ambiguity as to whether they are parents or not. Parents experiencing a stillbirth in a first pregnancy, Murphy argues, can question their very claim to parenthood whereas those experiencing stillbirth subsequent to the birth of a live child might still question the number of children they can claim to have, or have had. Central to this struggle with identity, the author concludes, is an ambiguity over the personhood of the stillborn baby which necessitates ambiguity over parental identification.

Chapter 10 by Linda Layne, draws on her long-term ethnographic research with pregnancy and infant loss support groups in the US. Layne uses the concepts of the 'canny' and 'uncanny' in this part of a larger project on emerging family forms including single mothers by choice and two-mom families, to examine how families deal with the absent presence of a member of the normative nuclear family. Specifically exploring the emergence of 'Angel Babies', Layne examines the practices of sexing, naming, picturing, and the creation of memorial baby dolls, arguing that these can be simultaneously both canny/uncanny, socially defiant/socially accepted and 'abnormal'/'normal'. She concludes by arguing that these practices sometimes make the strange more familiar, but at other times simply serve to accentuate the strangeness of reproductive loss.

The next two chapters explore the practice of memorialisation and consider changes to the expressions of private and public grief.

In Chapter 11, Kate Woodthorpe discusses the provision of baby gardens from the perspective of those who are tasked with providing and managing these spaces. In particular, she considers how they are managed, what takes place in these spaces, and how this is interpreted by cemetery staff. Woodthorpe draws on a series of interviews with individuals who work in cemeteries and crematoria to argue that the participants in her study saw the construction of baby gardens as creating a bounded community for lost babies and infants, akin to the metaphor of a 'nursery'. However, the author also argues that those responsible for managing baby gardens do so in a climate of rights whereby they are managing the expectations of grieving parents who desire to maintain personal continuing bonds with their dead children in what is ostensibly a public and managed space.

Chapter 12 also considers the practice of memorialisation following loss after stillbirth. However, in this chapter, Anna Davidsson Bremborg considers how internet memorialisation may be creating changed norms and values in both individualised and collective forms of grief and bereavement. Drawing on open data from a Swedish internet community site for parents bereaved by stillbirth, the author argues that the internet and new ways of grief go hand-in-hand. Whilst people who had experienced loss may have felt isolated in the past, Davidsson Bremborg argues that the internet affords these 'Angel Parents' the opportunity to share emotional feelings of grief, as well as stories about memorial ritualisation. These stories, the author concludes, have begun to change norms about what can be done and what is considered appropriate, or not when a baby dies within a global and increasingly connected world.

The final four chapters focus on that way that professionals understand reproductive loss, their performance at the boundary of life and death, and the way that this frames reproductive experiences.

In Chapter 13 Susannah Thompson maps changing understandings of perinatal loss in Australia in the twentieth and early twenty-first centuries. Here Thompson suggests that reproductive technologies as well as cultural understandings of grief and bereavement have changed over time and that these have influenced knowledge, understanding and practices surrounding the experiences of perinatal loss. At the beginning of the twentieth century, Thompson argues, pro-natalist ideology positioned perinatal loss as a form of (somewhat inevitable) 'foetal wastage' that threatened a healthy society. However, by the 1970s, miscarriage and stillbirth came to be seen as an individual loss whereby mothers, in particular, were seen in need of emotional support. More latterly, the author argues that the increasing use of prenatal technologies has increased the focus on maternal responsibility and on the expectation of positive pregnancy outcomes.

Jan Bleyen also uses a historical approach in Chapter 14. His focus is on the act of hiding or showing the stillborn child. Bleyen draws on open-ended qualitative interview data from retired and practising Flemish gynaecologists, midwives and pastors working in small hospital environments to show that the management of dead babies' bodies is an act of performing meanings of death and grief in ways that are both corporeal and sensory. Focusing predominantly on the oral history of a 57-year old retired Flemish midwife, Bleyen argues that death is made present through metaphor, and portrays a pessimistic image of past practices.

Chapter 15, written by Carol Komaromy questions the now popular Western practice of showing the dead baby to parents. However, here, the focus is on the emotional management of feelings in hospital settings in the UK following stillbirth and neonatal death. Komaromy draws on an interview with a midwife charged with the care of a woman who has experienced a stillbirth, and the account of a grandmother following the stillbirth of her grandson to interrogate the use of professional protocols designed to facilitate the grieving process. In this chapter Komaromy employs the sociological concepts of performativity and emotional labour to argue that those charged with the responsibility of caring for people who have experienced a stillbirth or neonatal death need to present a professional demeanour which involves the management of their own feelings. However, these individuals also provide the framework via which parents are given 'permission' to show their feelings. Komaromy argues that not all emotions are deemed as acceptable and the experience of loss is always assumed to be sad and painful, not allowing for the expression of ambivalence or other emotions. This new orthodoxy, she argues, can constrain the expression of authentic emotions that might be at odds with protocol and prescribed expectations.

In the final contribution to the book, Chapter 16 provides an analysis of four research projects that explored patient and professional views on feticide prior to termination of pregnancy for foetal anomaly, treatment withdrawal from sick neonates, and miscarriage in the UK. Using a broadly social constructionist approach, Ruth Graham, Nick Embleton, Allison Farnworth, Kathy Mason, Judith Rankin and Steve Robson consider issues of difference and diversity and the responses of various health professionals such as midwives, neonatologists, gynaecologists, nurses and others in responding to pregnancy loss. Echoing the views expressed by Komaromy in the previous chapter, Graham and colleagues argue for the use of discretion in reproductive health care and warn against structured responses, or 'best' practice, that can leave little room for bereaved parents to exercise their own agency.

Using this Book

We hope that whatever leads you to this book, that you find it useful and interesting. Our approach to reproductive loss, which we define broadly, means that we set ourselves quite a tall order in producing a book that represents all of this. We have done our best, but as with all such collections, there are omissions and there is room for continued reflection, writing and research in this field.

References

Earle, S., Foley, P., Komaromy, C. and Lloyd, C.E. 2008. Conceptualising reproductive loss: implications for understanding human fertility. *Human Fertility* [Online] 11(4), 259-262. Available at: http://dx.doi.org/10.1080/14647270802298272 [accessed: 3 February 2012].

Layne, L.L. 2003. Unhappy endings: a feminist reappraisal of the women's health movement from the vantage of pregnancy loss. *Social Science and Medicine*, 56: 1881-891.

Chapter 1

'Infertility' and 'Involuntary Childlessness': Losses, Ambivalences and Resolutions

Gayle Letherby

'Infertility' is a biological condition and 'involuntary childlessness' a social experience. Of course, it is possible to experience both; that is, a woman or man suffering from primary 'infertility' who is not parenting any children within a social relationship. However, it is also necessary to remember that people who are medically defined as 'infertile' may not wish necessarily to have children. Those who are medically 'infertile' may be parenting their biological children and wish to have more, yet the term 'involuntary childlessness' does not cover this experience, and those who are parenting their biological offspring following medical assistance may still be technically 'infertile'. In this chapter I draw on both my own and others' research findings to reflect further on the differences (and similarities) between 'infertility' and 'involuntary childlessness' both problematic terms as I will show.

In the 1990s I conducted a study into how issues of 'infertility' and 'involuntary childlessness' were defined in relation to identity.[1] My interest in this work originated in my own miscarriage, 'infertility' and non-motherhood and my research is focused on this auto/biographical experience. I felt that the losses associated with these events and experiences were both misunderstood and under-researched and during the process of data collection I came across many others who felt the same. Auto/biography – focusing on one, several or multiple lives – highlights the need to liberate the individual from individualism; to demonstrate how individuals are social selves. Furthermore, a focus on the individual can contribute to the understanding of the general (Mills 1959, Stanley 1992, Evans 1997). Auto/biographical work also highlights the relationship(s) and similarities

1 Using qualitative methods – single and dyad interviews and research by correspondence – with 65 women and eight men my study group included parents achieved through unaided biological conception, as a result of assisted conception, through adoption and step-parenthood and non-parents. The majority, but not all, had undergone tests and/or some medical treatment which related to their 'infertility'/childlessness. Twenty of the 65 women were mothers: 12 biologically (five following medical assistance) and eight socially; ages range from early 20s to early 70s. As well as these differences of experience and age, different economic groupings were also represented. There were some differences that were not represented; for example respondents were predominantly white and predominantly heterosexual.

and differences between the self and other within the research and writing process (Morgan 1998).

Motherhood and fatherhood are often taken for granted aspects of auto/biography: an inevitable identity within an individual's lifecourse. So when social circumstances and physical conditions prevent this the result is often distress (see Letherby 1994, Exley and Letherby 2001, Allison 2010, Greil et al. 2010). Thus, while the terms 'infertility' and 'involuntary childlessness' rightly imply losses and absences, experience is often more complex than these labels suggest. In consideration of this complexity these terms and other issues and concepts such as desperation, exclusion, ambivalence and resolution are discussed and critiqued.

Definitions

In contemporary western societies more women (and couples) choose to remain childless and there are higher numbers of 'infertility' cases than ever before. Those who have children do so later and have less. Increasing numbers of babies are born following some form of 'assistance': from self-administered donated sperm to medically sophisticated procedures. As Lorraine Culley et al. (2009, p.1) note '[d]ifferences in definitions, measurement criteria and healthcare systems between countries make global estimates of the prevalence of "infertility" difficult'. This problem of definition is extended to research populations as Greil et al (2010: 142) argues:

> In most studies, infertile individuals are implicitly and inadvertently defined operationally as 'people who present themselves for infertility treatment'. Once we move beyond treatment seekers we observe that the line between infertile and non-infertile people becomes blurred and infertile individuals are seen to constitute a much more diverse group than was previously understood.

Greil et al. (2010) suggest that those suffering from 'infertility' extend beyond the clinic and if you include 'involuntary childlessness' the population is much greater. Loss, ambivalence and adaptation characterises all of these experiences not least because of the significance of the identities of motherhood and fatherhood.

In 1981 Oakley argued that for many women children represented their main possibility of achievement and power and with colleagues in 1994, she added that 'choice' in this area for women is something of a misnomer given societal expectations. Contemporaneously, Coppock et al. (1995) suggested that women's 'rightful' role as mothers has been espoused historically as 'natural' by virtue of their capacity to bear children: motherhood is a 'rite of passage', invariably equated with 'womanhood' and glorified as women's chief vocation. Thus, many writers continue to argue that motherhood is key to women's identity in a way that fatherhood is not to men's (Letherby 1994, McAllister with Clarke 1998, Letherby and Williams 1999, Gillespie 2000, Wilson 2007):

> For many people, 'childless' implies a person with something missing from her (sic) life. Mothers are perceived as 'proper' women, while women without children are perceived as 'improper' and treated as 'other'. They are also treated as childlike rather than fully adult. Thus, women who have no children are considered to have no responsibilities and thus to be like children themselves (Letherby and Williams 1999: 723).

While the identity of mother has always been closely identified with caring and nurturing, fatherhood traditionally has been linked to the biological: the father as the provider of seed is significant in terms of genetic ties and family lines (Walker 1985, Katz Rothman 1988). Also, fathers have been associated with power, authority and status and it seems to follow that good fathers are good providers. This implies that the biological aspect of fatherhood and the patriarchal status are important for men and masculine identity, but other social and emotional elements of fathering such as caring and nurturing are less important. Yet, despite the continued focus on men as providers, both of sperm and money, contemporary fathers are expected to and desire more involved fatherhood (e.g. Brannen and Nilsen 2006, Dermont 2008, Fletcher and St George 2011).

As noted earlier, in addition to those who have been defined as medically 'infertile' – unable to carry a baby to term or unable to get pregnant after one year of trying – 'involuntary childlessness' can be the result of social rather than physical circumstances. This group can include among others; individuals whose children have died, those whose children are taken away from them or who lose custody cases, birth parents who give their children up for adoption and those who never meet someone with whom they want to parent or have a desire to parent that their partner does not share. I reflect on some of these and other childless experiences in the remainder of this chapter.

Reflecting on Losses and Absences

As Pfeffer and Woollett (1983: 82) suggest '[it] seems that once you find yourself involuntarily childless, all other identifying marks are washed away'. Such transformations are not unusual; they are the hallmark of socially stigmatizing conditions Goffman 1963). With specific reference to 'infertility' and 'involuntary childlessness' the dominant discourses of social loss, biological identity and medial hope in contemporary academic and 'scientific' publications all operate to give a picture that supports the dominant social order (Franklin 1990). It is not surprising then that people in this situation feel less than normal, as data from my 1997 study suggests:

> Life as a parent and mother is wonderful. It somehow becomes normal. You become part of the world instead of detached from it (Abi).

> People can tell by looking at me that I am handicapped. A failure to womankind. I feel like half a woman (Tracey).

> It felt like a loss of manhood. I felt stripped of something I was expected to do. I am the last in the male line. Someone asked me once 'is your semen different?' I don't know 'is it?' It bothered me for a while [pause]. Yes it bothered me … I felt a lot less of a man (Will).

There is evidence that undergoing 'infertility treatment' and deciding to stop treatment can add to the distress individuals feel. Thus, the experience of treatment can be stressful and distressing in itself (see for example Franklin 1990, Thosby 2004, Allison 2010). Many women and couples feel a sense of loss each time, following a treatment cycle, a pregnancy is not achieved or achieved and lost and the decision to stop treatment involves a transition from 'not yet pregnant' to 'not going to be pregnant' (Thosby 2004: 162). Again my data confirm this:

> You've got to have it if it's there. But then your sense of failure is greater if it doesn't work (Kate).

> … they said I had a good chance. I built up my hopes and then felt bad when it didn't work. You've got to stop somewhere and realise that you are not going to have … Treatment is a good thing as long as you are willing to give up (Emily).

A plethora of research highlights the stigma and pity that is conferred on women and men who are childless – whether by choice or through social or physical reasons (see Franklin 1990, Letherby 1999, 2002; Thosby 2004). Sometimes however, because male 'infertility' is often associated with virility and 'manhood' (see Will's account above), hostile humour is directed at childless men instead (Exley and Letherby 2001). The negative responses of others meant individuals and couples sometimes concealed their reasons for childlessness:

> Phil and I had decided not to discuss our apparent infertility with anyone as this, we felt, would make it less stressful for us. I didn't want people to keep asking if we had any 'news' yet or looking closely at my waistline.

> I can't really explain why I didn't want to be more open about our infertility but some of the factors involved were 1. It was very personal and really involved just Phil and myself. 2. Didn't want people fussing and gossiping about us. 3. Didn't want sympathy. 4. Being open about it was rather like admitting defeat, we still had hope. (Rachel).

In his book on *Family Secrets* Bradshaw (1995) sites 'birth-related' secrets – i.e. those related to adoption, illegitimacy and infertility – as one of a group of 'dark secrets'. But managing disclosure, as did my respondents Rachel and Phil, can be one way of coping with 'infertility' – related loss in which Crawshaw (2010: 71) includes:

- control over destiny
- control of body function
- genetic continuity
- future as a biological mother or father
- future as a biological parent with partner
- physical experience of pregnancy, birth and early infancy
- fertile identity as an individual and/or as a couple
- providing a biological child for one's kinship system.

Clearly, people in these situations have constrained reproductive choices (Petchesky 1980). As Frannie, a study participant, explained:

> A 'woman's right to choose' has no relevance to my life, or many other women's and sometimes it feels as though that's the worse thing about infertility – not having a choice.

If 'infertility' and 'infertility treatments' lead to feelings of loss of control, adoption, which often follows 'infertility' treatment, can compound these feelings (Thorn 2010). Although, the recent rise in inter-racial celebrity adoptions may lead to greater acceptance of transracial adoptive families, internet adoption sites reveal assumptions that prospective adoptive parents wish for a child to whom others will assume they are genetically connected (Letherby and Marchbank 2003). The significance of kinship and the biological tie (Strathern 1992) and the fear of 'genetic death' (Houghton and Houghton 1984) are demonstrated partly by the rise of surrogacy, posthumous use of sperm to 'father' children and the purchasing of gametes. Biological (and if at all possible genetic) parenthood complement dominant discourses of 'true' motherhood and fatherhood and 'proper' families (see Letherby 1999, Culley et al. 2009). Adoptive parents have to 'accept the unknown'; a child or children with whom they have no genetic heritage, have not 'created' themselves and about whom they may know little (Thorn 2010). Additionally, in contemporary adoptions, some link with the birth family is often maintained which means that adoptive parents are continually reminded that their child/ren has another set of parents with whom they have a genetic relationship (Feast 2010). Some respondents were clear about their reasons for not considering this option:

> We haven't looked into adoption, I'm sure I'm too old anyway. We would rather selfishly like our own child (Pam).

> (T)he thought that one's children may turn out to be a disappointment, especially adopted ones as one doesn't know where they come from (Steph).

Of course, this is also true for those who opt for gamete donation (Murray and Golombok 2003, Freeman et al. 2009). Yet, despite concerns over 'genetic bewilderment' which can continue, even intensify as children grow (Thorn 2010), adoption and donor-assisted pregnancy often help feelings of 'infertility'-related loss (Letherby 2002, Feast 2010). Such was the case for many of the respondents in Julia Feast's 2005 study of adoptive parents, birth parents and adopted people. For example: 'Adopting our daughter helped me to overcome the sadness of not being able to have any further children myself.' 'Adopting a family satisfies all my longing to have children' (Feast 2010: 182).

Similarly, for a number of participants in this study childlessness was much more of an issue than genetic connection: '(N)o empty arms anymore. The need to mother is different from the need to give birth' (May). Alan and his wife had adopted two children and he was grateful not just for their children but for the access parenthood gave them to new social networks. Networks that he felt they had been excluded from previously: 'We have a completely different social life now we have the children. We go out much more.' But there are still gaps: 'How could I tell Tim about his birth? I wasn't there (Annie, adoptive mother).'

Arguably, recent public exposure of 'infertility' and 'involuntary childlessness' has added to the stigma of the condition. In addition, individuals and couples are judged as 'deserving' or 'undeserving' of 'infertility' treatment (Letherby 2003) and as appropriate or inappropriate biological or social parents (Minkoff and Ecker 2009, Crawshaw 2010). But feelings of loss associated with 'involuntary childlessness' are not new and there are many historical examples. As Nicholson (2007) reminds us the First World War led to the death of nearly three-quarters of a million British soldiers and, although many of these men left behind widows and orphans, many were unmarried when they died. Nicholson adds, 'Their deaths bereaved another generation: the thousands of women born, like them between 1885 and 1905, who unquestioningly believed marriage to be their birthright, only to have it snatched from them by four of the bloodiest years in human history' (2007: xiii). Two-thirds of older, unmarried women surveyed in the 1960s felt they had missed out on having children. Responses focused on the gaps that childlessness had left in their lives, the ways in which they felt reproached by others and their own feelings of failure (Nicholson 2007). Olive Wakeman born in 1907 and interviewed when aged 100 said, 'I would have loved to have had lots of children, and married, but I've got over that! (ibid: 122)'. Her way of coping with childlessness included immersing herself in childcare, as a nursery nurse and in caring for cousins and nephews and nieces. Similarly, Richmal Crompton, the author of over 40 volumes of the *Just William* books was reported to be a 'much loved aunt' (ibid: 124).

The identity of people whose children die before them is complex for, as Davidson and Stahls note: 'Mothers, however, remain mothers, not until the day their children die, but in experiential terms, until they themselves die, and in terms of family histories, even after their own deaths' (2010: 19).

Research suggests that those who have their children taken away, incarcerated parents and foster parents also experience significant grief (see Radosh 2002, Mullings 2010). Yet, they do not receive the sympathy that bereaved mothers and fathers do, whose grief is itself often silenced by others (Davidson and Stahls 2010). Likewise, the losses that birth parents who give up their child for adoption experience are often misunderstood or completely denied. Murray in her auto-ethnographic piece writes:

> If I had kept you, my baby, I would have been seen as a shameful, filthy, and worthless person but when I gave you up for adoption I was seen as selfish and uncaring (Lauderdale 1992). There was a perception from others that I would forget about you and move on. I never forgot you. However, I never let myself grieve openly as it was not socially acceptable at the time to speak of my unwed mothering experience (2010: 147).

Murray ends her piece:

> Our reunion brings with it an opportunity for healing and also a recognition of the enormity of the loss. But as I face my grief and shame and acknowledge it, I also realise that I am able to reclaim that part of myself that was lost (148).

Complex Identities

Alongside similar work, my research provides evidence that women and men without children represent the 'other' in a society that privileges parenthood above other attributes (e.g. Pfeffer and Woollett 1983, Franklin 1990, Nicholson 2007, Culley et al. 2009, Allison 2010). This can affect relationships with family, friends and partners negatively and 'infertile' and 'involuntarily childless' people often report feeling excluded. People who do not have children, and those who have achieved biological or social parenthood in 'different' ways, report feeling excluded in various situations: from the 'parenthood club', from discussions about pregnancy and birth, from their child's early life and/or an understanding of their genetic differences and so on (Letherby 1999, 2002, 2010a).

Such people not only have to live with their own losses and absences but also live with an identity which is different and often discredited or seen as lesser. As a result, many engage in considerable amounts of emotional self-management (Exley and Letherby 2001) and sometimes seek out the support of similar others and health and social care professionals to cope with their distress (see Greil et al. 2010 for a research review). External dominant representations and perceptions of 'infertile' and 'involuntarily childless' people are of 'desperate individuals' but the reality is often more complicated (Pfeffer and Woollett 1983, Franklin 1990, Letherby 1999, 2002). Although some respondents told me of their desperation about their 'infertility' and/or childlessness this was only one aspect of their identity and many had otherwise fulfilling lives. For some, this experience was the worst thing that had ever happened to them, for others it was not (Letherby 1999, 2002, 2010a). Despite much research highlighting the ambivalence of the actual and perceived experience and status of motherhood (e.g. de Beauvoir 1949, Hollway and Featherstone 1997, Gordon et al. 2005), less is concerned with ambivalence about 'infertility' and 'involuntary (and voluntary) childlessness'. My study participants were aware of the negative as well as the positive aspects of parenthood. Gloria who was childless said, 'I don't want to be solely so and so's mum. You lose some of your identity that way. Even if we had adopted, or had biological children. I would still want time for myself.' And Kate who became pregnant twice after low-level 'infertility' treatment but was unable to get pregnant again following more treatment said, 'I don't think of myself primarily as a mother, I think of myself as Kate. I have roles as a mother and a person who's looking for a job and a friend, wife, sister.'

Such feelings of ambivalence are not new:

> Winifred Holtby was robust about her childlessness. She did not deny her strong maternal feelings towards small children, but neither did she indulge in sentimental regrets for the babies she would never bear. [she was] forthright and realistic about children. Babies were 'a nuisance', and boring, and anyone considering having one should contemplate seriously the prospect of a great deal of laundry. At the same time she sought contact with them (Nicholson 2007: 125).

Tonkin (2010) writes of what she refers to as the disenfranchised grief of women who have 'left it too late' and thus suffer from unintentional childlessness. She coins the term 'contingently childless' to define 'women who have always seen themselves as having children but find themselves at the end of their natural fertility without having done so for social rather than (at least initially) medical reasons' (Tonkin 2010: 178). Tonkin (2010) adds that these women's feelings of loss may not be recognised by others or even articulated by themselves. There is yet another group whose grief may be silenced.

On reflection, the losses represented here are to some extent minimised, after all how is it possible to grieve for what one has never had? Yet, this chapter also highlights the intense feelings of loss experienced by many of those identified as 'infertile' or 'involuntarily childless' in societies that view parenthood as natural and inevitable. On the other hand, Szewczuk (first published online 2011) in her analysis of what she terms 'age-related infertility', that is 'infertility that is an outcome of fertility postponement' suggests that the rise in such cases offers a challenge to pro-natalist explanations. Postponement, she adds, was more common historically than we think, but the reliability of modern contraception results in 'a tale of two technologies' as it enables 'fertility to be put on the back burner, undiscussed; this delay leading in turn to age-related fertility problems and consequently to assisted conception' (2011). Clearly, time as well as ambivalence characterise reproductive 'choices' and experiences. Not just the 'right time' or not to have children but also the treatment takes time and time is a concept that can run out (Earle and Letherby 2007).

Time is also relevant to any consideration of resolution. One motivation for this research was my frustration at readings that implied the only resolutions possible were to achieve parenthood or accept childlessness. From my data, I suggest that adaptation, rather than resolution, is a more appropriate term for, as the life course continues, new adjustments are necessary to the loss of grandparenthood (as well as parenthood); the development of a child whose genetic origins are different; being reunited with one's birth child; one's changing feelings and where people locate themselves on the 'involuntary' – 'voluntary' childless continuum (Monach 1993, Woollett 1996).

Final Thoughts

Increasing 'infertility' and 'childlessness' is perceived as a loss to society as well as a loss to an individual or couple's own auto/biography. For example, across Europe there are currently concerns about below replacement fertility:

> As birthrates continue to decline or, in some cases, increase slightly, nevertheless to remain below replacement level … politicians, demographers and policy-makers alike grapple with fears about "demographic crises," "birth strikes," the "death of the nation," and "baby busts." Simultaneously, Europe's populations are graying, straining pension and health systems. To address projected demographic dramas associated with declining birthrates, Europe's leaders – supranational, national and local – are proposing various strategies ranging from female and family-friendly pronatalist policies to targeted immigration and return migration (Kligman 2005: 249).

As Kligman (2005) adds, the discourses about demographic crisis reflect particular views about who 'should' and invoke categories of otherness in that they 'simultaneously signify that the nation's "proper" inhabitants are not producing whereas its "others" are reproducing too much' (Kligman 2005: 253).

Therefore, 'infertility' and 'involuntary childlessness' is not just a personal or couple experience but one that is influenced by and commented on by external others. The status and experience associated with these identities is complex and varied as are the related losses, ambivalences and resolutions. Reflecting on her own changing identity with reference to her work on 'infertility' and 'involuntary childlessness' Woollett notes:

> … my perspective on infertility has changed from that of 'insider' to that of 'Other', but coming as I have to this perspective from the position of 'insider', it is probably more appropriate to position myself as experienced or privileged

> 'Other', thereby raising questions about the usefulness of the insider/outsider dualism (1996: 71).

I appreciate and agree with this in terms of my position. I also believe that my own experience of loss, ambivalence and resolution owes much to other opportunities that I have had. As I have written elsewhere:

> … my desires and intentions have been subject to change and even though I am aware of the constraints on my 'choice' it feels like a choice nevertheless. Twenty-six years? ago when I had my miscarriage my central aim was to be a mother and I felt that I was only half a woman without a child. Any doubts or ambivalences I had about becoming a mother I denied. Now I feel very different. I no longer feel a lesser woman (or less than adult) for not mothering children. I am also able to accept the equivocal nature of my desires – that is, a part of me enjoys the freedom that I have had and have because of my biologically childless state. If I had become a biological mother I know that I would have felt opposing emotions in relation to that experience also.

Now self-defining as more (biologically) 'voluntarily childless' than 'involuntarily childless' I credit this shift in part to the opportunities my academic endeavours have given me for detailed reflection on my own experience and those of similar others: an opportunity that most people do not have (Letherby 2010b: 264-265).

References

Allison, J. 2010. Grieving Conceptions: making motherhood in the wake of infertility in Ireland. *Journal of the Motherhood Initiative for Research and Community Involvement*, 1(2), 219-231.

Brannen, J. and Nilsen, A. 2006. From Fatherhood to Fathering: transmission and change among British fathers in four generation families. *Sociology*, 40(2), 335-352.

Bradshaw, J. 1995. *Family Secrets: What you don't know can hurt you*. New York: Bantham Books.

Coppock, V. Haydon, D. and Richter, I. 1995. *The Illusions of 'Post Feminism': new women, old myths*. London: Taylor and Francis.

Crawshaw. M. 2010. Assessing Infertility Couple for Adoption: just what does 'coming to terms with infertility' mean? in *Adopting After Infertility: messages for practice, research and personal experience*, edited by M. Crawshaw and R. Balen. London: Jessica Kingsley, 68-88.

Culley L. Hudson, N. and Van Rooij, F. 2009. Introduction: Ethnicity, Infertility and Assisted Reproductive Technologies in *Marginalized Reproduction: Ethnicity, infertility and reproductive technologies*, edited by L. Culley, N. Hudson and F. Van Rooij. London: Earthscan, 1-14.

Davidson, D. and Stahls, H. 2010. Maternal Grief: creating an environment for dialogue. *Journal of the Motherhood Initiative for Research and Community Involvement*, 1(2), 16-25.

de Beauvoir, S. 1949. *The Second Sex* (translated by H. M. Parshley, Penguin 1972).

Dermott, E. 2008. *Intimate Fatherhood.* London: Routledge.

Earle, S. and Letherby, G. 2007. Conceiving Time?: Women who do or do not conceive. *Sociology of Health and Illness*, 29(2), 233-250.

Evans, M. 1997. *Introducing Contemporary Feminist Thought.* Cambridge: Polity Press.

Exley, C. and Letherby, G. 2001. Managing a Disrupted Lifecourse: issues of identity and emotion work. *Health*, 5(1), 112-31.

Feast, J. 2010. Infertility and Adoption: the search for birth parents and the impact on adult family relationships in *Adopting After Infertility: messages for practice, research and personal experience* edited by M. Crawshaw and R. Balen. London: Jessica Kingsley, 180-193.

Fletcher, R. and StGeorge, J. 2011. Heading into fatherhood-nervously: support for fathering from online dads. *Qualitative Health Research*, 28(8), 1101-1114.

Franklin, S. 1990. Deconstructing 'Desperateness': The social construction of infertility in popular representations of new reproductive technologies in *The New Reproductive Technologies*, edited by M.V. McNeil and S. Yearley. Hampshire and London: Macmillan, 200-229.

Freeman, T. Jadva, V. Kramer, W. and Golombok, W. 2009. Gamete donation: parents' experiences of searching for their child's donor siblings and donor. *Human Reproduction*, 24(3), 505-516.

Gillespie, R. 2000. When No Means No: disbelief, disregard and deviance as discourses of voluntary childlessness. *Women's Studies International Forum*, 23(2), 223-234.

Goffman, E. 1963. *Stigma: Notes on the Management of Spoiled Identity.* Harmondsworth: Penguin.

Gordon, T. Holland, J. Lahelma, E. and Thomson, R. 2005. Imagining Gendered Adulthood: Anxiety, Ambivalence, Avoidance and Anticipation. *European Journal of Women's Studies*, 12(1), 83-103.

Greil, A.L. Slauson-Blevins, K, McQuillan, J. 2010. The Experience of Infertility: a review of recent literature. *Sociology of Health and Illness*, 32(1), 140-162.

Hollway, W. and Featherstone, B. 1997. *Mothering and Ambivalence.* London: Routledge.

Houghton, D. and Houghton, P. 1984. *Coping with Childlessness.* London: Unwin Hyman.

Katz Rothman, B. 1988. *The Tentative Pregnancy: Prenatal diagnosis and the future of motherhood.* London: Pandora.

Kligman, G. 2005. A Reflection on Barren States: the demographic paradoxes of consumer capitalism, in *Barren States: the population 'implosion' in Europe*, edited by C.B. Douglass. Oxford: Berg, 249-260.

Letherby, G. 1994. Mother or Not, Mother or What?: problems of definition and identity. *Women's Studies International Forum*, 17(5), 525-532.

Letherby, G. 1999. Other than Mother and Mothers as Others: the experience of motherhood and non-motherhood in relation to 'infertility' and 'involuntary childlessness'. *Women's Studies International Forum*, 22(3), 359-372.

Letherby, G. 2000. Dangerous Liaisons: auto/biography in research and research writing, in *Danger in the Field: risk and ethics in social research*, edited by G. Lee-Treweek and S. Linkogle. London: Routledge, 91-113.

Letherby, G. 2002. Challenging Dominant Discourses: identity and change and the experience of 'infertility' and 'involuntary childlessness.' *Journal of Gender Studies*, 11(3), 277-288.

Letherby, G. 2003. Battle of the Gametes: cultural representation of medically assisted conception, in *Gender, Identity and Reproduction: social perspectives*, edited by S. Earle and G. Letherby. London: Palgrave, 50-65.

Letherby, G. 2010a. When treatment ends, in *Adopting after Infertility: Messages from practice, research and personal experience*, edited by M. Crawshaw and R. Balen. London: Jessica Kingsley Publishers, 29-42.

Letherby, G. 2010b. Reflecting on Loss as a M/Other and a Feminist Sociologist. *Journal of the Motherhood Initiative for Research and Community Involvement*, 1(2), 258-269.

Letherby, G. and Marchbank, J. 2002. Cyber-chattels: buying brides and babies on the net, in *Dot.cons: crime, deviance and identity on the internet*, edited by Y. Jewkes. Devon: Willan, 68-85.

Letherby, G. and Williams, C. 1999. Non-motherhood: ambivalent autobiographies. *Feminist Studies*, 25(3), 719-728.

McAllister, F. and Clarke, L. 1988. *Choosing Childlessness*. London: Family Policy Studies Centre.

Mills, C.W. 1959 [1970]. *The Sociological Imagination.* London: Penguin.

Minkoff, H. and Ecker, J. 2009. The California octuplets and the duties of reproductive endocrinologists. *American Journal of Obstetrics and Gynecology*, 201(1), 15.e1-15.e3. Available at: http://www.ajog.org/article/S0002-9378(09)00489-X [accessed: 26 March 2012].

Monach, J.H. 1993. *Childless No Choice: the experience of involuntary childlessness.* London: Routledge.

Morgan, D. 1998. Sociological Imaginations and Imagining Sociologies: bodies, auto/biographies and other mysteries. *Sociology*, 32(4), 647-63.

Mullings, D.V. 2010. Temporary Mothering: grieving the loss of foster children when they leave. *Journal of the Motherhood Initiative for Research and Community Involvement*, 1(2), 165-176.

Murray, C. and Golombok, S. 2003. To Tell Or Not To Tell: The decision-making process of egg-donation parents. *Human Fertility*, 6(2), 89-95.

Murray, L. 2010. Secrets of an 'Illegitimate' Mom. *Journal of the Motherhood Initiative for Research and Community Involvement*, 1(2), 139-149.

Nicholson, V. 2007. *Singled Out.* London: Penguin.

Oakley, A. 1981. *Subject Women.* Oxford: Martin Robinson.
Petchesky, R.P. 1980. Reproductive Freedom: beyond 'a woman's right to choose'. *Signs: Journal of Women in Culture and Society*, 5(66), 661-685.
Pfeffer, N. and Woollett, A. 1983. *The Experience of Infertility.* London: Virago.
Radosh, P.F. 2002. Reflections on Women's Crime and Mothers in Prison: A peacemaking approach. *Crime and Delinquency*, 48(2), 300-315.
Stanley, L. 1992. *The Auto/biographical I: The Theory and Practice of Feminist auto/biography.* Manchester University Press: Manchester.
Strathern, M. 1992. *After Nature: English Kinship in the Late Twentieth Century.* Cambridge: Cambridge University Press.
Szewczuk, E. 2012. Age-related infertility: a tale of two technologies. *Sociology of Health and Illness*, 34(3), 429-443.
Thorn, P. 2010. The shift from medical treatment to adoption: Exploring family building options, in *Adopting after Infertility: Messages from Practice, Research and Personal Experience*, edited by M. Crawshaw and R. Balen, London: Jessica Kingsley Publishers, 43-54.
Thosby, K. 2004. *When IVF Fails: feminism, infertility and the negotiation of normality.* Houndmills: Palgrave Macmillan.
Tonkin, L. 2010. Making Sense of Loss: the 'disenfranchised grief of women who are 'contingently childless'. *Journal of the Motherhood Initiative for Research and Community Involvement*, 1(2), 177-187.
Walker, M. 1985. *Alone of All Her Sex: The myth and cult of the Virgin Mary.* London: Picador.
Wilson, S. 2007. 'When you have children, you're obliged to live': motherhood, chronic illness and biographical disruption. *Sociology of Health and Illness*, 29(4), 610-626.
Woollett, A. 1996. Infertility: from inside/out to outside/in, in *Representing the Other: a feminism and psychology reader*, edited by S. Wilkinson and C. Kitzinger. London: Sage.

Chapter 2

International Perspectives on the Sterilization of Women with Intellectual Disabilities

Liz Tilley, Jan Walmsley, Sarah Earle and Dorothy Atkinson

The literature on human reproduction has, with some notable exceptions, ostensibly ignored the experiences of people with intellectual disabilities. Reproductive rights have been central to much feminist social sciences literature in this field and the right of women to 'control their own bodies' remains the cornerstone of this debate (see Petchesky 1986). Whilst some commentators have extended this to include the experiences of disabled women (see Morris 1996) disability is most often featured in the context of new reproductive technologies (see Shaw 2004) and so the experiences of disabled women have remained outside of mainstream debate.

In this chapter we focus on the sterilization of women with intellectual disabilities. We offer an international perspective, although one which draws predominantly on evidence from modern western societies, with a special focus on the UK context. In part it is a historical review, since the practice of involuntary sterilization is now subject to strict legal regulation. However, despite developments in Human Rights and Mental Capacity legislation, lack of control over contraceptive and reproductive choices continues to feature in the lives of women with intellectual disabilities. While the mass involuntary sterilization of women with intellectual disabilities is no longer a feature of current policy and practice in western societies, other forms of reproductive control – notably the use of long-term contraception such as Depo Provera[1] – appear to be commonly used. In this chapter we draw upon the authors' interests in oral history, life story approaches, social policy and health sociology to explore this hidden area of reproductive loss.

1 Depo-Provera (medroxyprogesterone acetate) is an injectable medicine that prevents conception for up to 3 months with each injection. It works by preventing the ovarian egg cells from maturing and releasing from the ovary.

A Short History of Sterilization

There is a long and dishonourable history of sterilizing women with intellectual disabilities in western societies. In the early twentieth century, the practice of sterilizing women without their consent was legalized by statute in the majority of US states, in two Canadian provinces, in Sweden, Iceland, Switzerland, Austria, Denmark and Norway. It was mooted seriously in the UK in the 1930s; in 1934 the recommendation of the departmental Committee on Sterilisation (most commonly referred to as the Brock Committee) was *not* to legalize sterilization without consent (see Thomson 1998 for a detailed discussion). Legislation permitting sterilization remained on the statute books of many countries until the 1970s but it now has been largely abandoned.

The literature suggests that the sterilization of women with intellectual disabilities stemmed from the belief that 'mental defect' was inherited (Jones 1986, Laughlin 1926, reprinted 2004, Reilly 1977). It is thus explicitly associated with the era of eugenics. For example, Park and Radford cite a post-World War 2 Canadian paper entitled 'Sterilise the Unfit' in which they argued that:

> The free propagation of mental subnormals is carrying us far in the direction of race deterioration (Hincks 1946 quoted in Park and Radford 1998: 319).

Sterilization was only one weapon in the armoury of eugenicists in the UK (and elsewhere). The fear that people with intellectual disabilities would reproduce was also the driving force behind the segregated institutionalization of people with intellectual disabilities (Jackson 2000). The 1913 Mental Deficiency Act in England and Wales required Local Authorities to place people in institutions if they were deemed 'feeble minded', 'morally defective', 'imbeciles' or 'idiots'. Eventually, this resulted in the creation of large institutions, in which people were housed, with strict segregation of the sexes designed to prevent men and women having sexual intercourse. Those people who avoided institutionalization were supervised in the community and many lived with their family. Minute and detailed scrutiny of homes was part of the role of Mental Deficiency Visitors in the inter-war period; Visitors (mostly women) usually worked in a voluntary capacity and their role included the provision of family support, as well as surveillance (Walmsley and Rolph 2001). Visitors were required to complete documentation which included the question: '(f) Is it considered that the control available would prevent the defective from procreating children?' (Board of Control Model Form 1929) For authorities mindful of expense, it was tempting to regard sterilization as a relatively inexpensive way of discharging their obligation to prevent people with intellectual disabilities from conceiving, and there is clear evidence of English Local Authorities campaigning for such legislation at the end of the 1920s (Fennell 1996).

The English Board of Control archives show that child-rearing was of greater concern when people with intellectual disabilities were married, as being married allowed couples to keep their children (Board of Control Annual Report 1926).

These sentiments were echoed at a local level, as shown by research in the English county of Somerset. The local Mental Deficiency Committee argued that if a known defective young woman was married then the Committee could not exercise its powers under the Mental Deficiency Act. This afforded the possibilty that she could go on to have a large family, which would be prevented if controlled in an institutional setting. As such, the Committee pressed for changes in the law through the introduction of certificates of fitness before marriage that could prevent mentally defective people from marrying in the first place (Fennell 1996).

However, as we argue in this chapter and elsewhere (Tilley et al. 2012), it is a mistake to regard sterilization as a mere historical aberration. Arguably, the credibility of scientific eugenicism waned following the Holocaust, but sterilization continued to be practised extensively in many countries after the discrediting of Nazi ideals, well into the 1970s. Instead, sterilization became reframed as being of social and therapeutic benefit (Dyer 1987, Thomson 1998), ideas which still persist today and carry unfortunate consequences for women's rights and reproductive choice.

Sterilization and Institutions

Much of the evidence concerning historical sterilization practices in the international context relates to institutions. In a number of those jurisdictions where it was legal to impose involuntary sterilization it appears to have become routine to sterilize inmates, mostly women, though in both California (Edgerton 1967) and Alberta (Park and Radford 1998) men were also sterilized. Indeed, in both California and Alberta it appears that sterilization was practiced on most if not all (female and male) residents (Edgerton 1967, Park and Radford 1998). In an interview recorded in 2010, Leilani Muir, who had been an inmate of the Provincial Training School in Red Deer, Alberta, recalled that she was subjected to a routinized practice:

> I was taken to the clinic. I was told when I got there that I was going to have my appendix out. I wasn't in any pain, but I was just doing what I was told. There was four of us who had the surgery the same day. I did not know that my life would be ruined for the rest of my life that day (Open University on i-Tunes U, 2010).

In Sweden and Iceland, sterilization appears to have been a prerequisite for discharge from institutions and also fairly routinized (Stefansdóttir and Hreinsdóttir 2011). Kristina Engwall's (2004) research into Vastra Mark in Sweden indicates that undergoing voluntary sterilization was a condition of women being released, and notes that out of 481 medical case files '15.. explicitly reported that the patient objected to sterilization. However, if not consenting meant remaining in the institution, it can hardly be termed "voluntary"' (2004: 89). Ragnheiður, an Icelandic woman who had been institutionalised in the late twentieth century recalled:

> It is so strange. When I moved to the group home I had to undergo sterilization. I didn't agree but I had to agree because otherwise I would not be allowed to move from the institution (Stefansdóttir and Hreinsdóttir 2011).

Ladd Taylor (2004), writing about Minnesota, also indicates that agreement to being sterilized enabled women to stay out of instutitions, and that this was fiscally driven, to save the cost of an institutional place.

Most of the historical evidence relating to the sterilization of women with intellectual disabilities is from institutions, and countries and states where involuntary sterilization was legally sanctioned. Formally, mass sterilizations of people with intellectual disabilities practised legally ended in the 1970s when the legislation was repealed. Next we explore the much less well-documented evidence of sterilization practice in the community.

Sterilization Outside Institutions

In the UK, legislation sanctioning the involuntary sterilization of women with intellectual disabilities was never passed.[2] However, this does not mean that sterilization was not practised before 1988, only that it was not routinely documented and emergent oral history evidence indicates that sterilization was not uncommon. People were frequently deceived about what was going to happen, for example, Ebba Hreinsdóttir, whose mother agreed to have her sterilized at the age of 14, was told she was to have her appendix removed, just like Leilani Muir in Canada.

Although evidence is extremely limited, some individuals in the UK were apparently encouraged to undergo sterilization following institutional discharge. Irene, interviewed by Walmsley in 1991, recalled this series of events following discharge from a long stay hospital. We estimate the date of the operation to be mid 1970s:

---

2 Prior to 1988 it was unclear whether it was lawful or unlawful to sterilize a woman over the age of 18 who was deemed 'non compos mentos' and could not give her consent to the procedure. Whilst the courts did have some powers regarding sterilization decisions relating to minors, there was no power, in statute or common law, for the courts to sanction the procedure when the person reached the age of 18 if that person could not give consent (TheMentalWeb.com 2011). Professionals undertaking the procedure ran the risk of being accused of medical battery. Following the case of Re F, it was set down in common law that court approval would be required before any such procedure for contraceptive reasons took place; and that approval would only be granted as a last resort and in the best interests of the patient, to guard against sterilization being performed for the sake of convenience. See http://www.thementalweb.com/index.php/caselaw/cases-pre-2009/93-re-f-mental-patient-sterilisation-1990-2-ac-1-hl.html for a detailed account of this case.

> Then I went in Luton and Dunstable Hospital, operation, sterilized.
>
> …
>
> Long while ago Mr. Brennan down the Centre, he says 'Irene, you don't want a baby'. Mr. Brennan went up there; he said 'I don't want Irene to have that baby'. Took me in the clinic, test me. Yeh, I'm all right, I'm on pills. Oh God, God, tempers, throwing things. I can't remember him, I can't remember anybody, it's those tablets. When I went in the clinic me blood pressure went up high. You know what it was, it's them pills. I'm not taking them no more. Then they took me in the hospital, then I'm all right. Yeah, Doctor Hamilton operated, 10 hours I was underneath (Walmsley 1991 unpublished interview transcript).

One could not say that Irene was deceived, indeed she appeared to welcome the opportunity to be sterilized, and to come off the contraceptive pill. When she was interviewed she was in a long-term relationship with a man, and apparently enjoying her sex life. The apparent informality of the process Irene described is striking. Its very normality is indicated by this chance comment by a member of a UK women's group: 'People like us don't have babies. No one in the centre does apart from staff. Some people have their stomachs taken out' (Atkinson and Williams 1990: 175).

Evidence suggests that sterilization may have been quite common in England until relatively recently. A survey undertaken in England c.1990 found that over half of 274 responding family members would have or had considered sterilization for their child (Bambrick and Roberts 1991, quoted in Stansfield, Holland Clare 2007: 35). Roy et al.'s study (1993) found that alternative contraception had not been explored by family members considering sterilization (quoted in Stansfield 2007: 36). The most recent research study on the subject in England and Wales was a detailed review of 73 applications for sterilization which went before the Official Solicitor between 1988 and 1999 (Stansfield, Holland Clare 2007). Under mental capacity legislation in England and Wales (Mental Capacity Act 2005), sterilization is only lawful if an individual has the mental capacity to consent. If he or she lacks capacity there has to be a formal application to the court for contraceptive purposes. If sterilization is considered to be for 'therapeutic' purposes however, and in the best interests of the person, an application may not be needed (Stansfield 2007). The Court must be satisfied that the individual is unable to consent, and that the sterilization is in their best interests because of likelihood of pregnancy, the probable risks of pregnancy and parenthood (psychological damage) and the efficacy of alternative contraception.

Seventy of the cases examined by Stansfield, Holland and Clare (2007) were women, three were men, and 37 per cent were minors. The average age of the women in question was 21.4 years. Of these:

- 75 per cent were not in established relationships
- 21 (29 per cent) were known to be sexually active
- 86 per cent had never been pregnant
- 25 per cent were probably the victims of sexual abuse – in 9 cases sexual abuse was documented, in a further 9 non-consensual sexual activity was suspected
- More than a third were using recognized chemical or mechanical contraception
- A third of women were subjected to supervision as a method of contraception.

Thirty-one sterilizations were approved, 28 of these were tubal ligation, and three were hysterectomies. Six procedures went ahead without the need for court approval because the procedure was deemed 'therapeutic', the procedure purporting significant physical, psychological and/or social benefits. Thus, roughly half the cases that were considered were deemed suitable for sterilization.

Stansfield, Holland and Clare (2007) explored UK case records from 1988 until 1999; but there is very little evidence on practices after this period, despite the implementation of the Mental Capacity Act 2005 in England and Wales which in principle provides a new framework for decision-making in relation to reproductive rights. However, there is some recent evidence about practice in the past ten years from other western countries. For example, a Belgian study of 397 women aged 18-46 found that 22 per cent had been sterilized (Servais et al. 2004), and a Dutch study involving 397 women aged 15-59 of whom 112 were using contraception, found that 25 had been sterilized, 20 of these prior to 2000 (van Schrojenstein Lantman-de Valk, Rooks and Maaskant 2011). Under New Zealand law people with intellectual disabilities may be sterilized, without their consent, and court authorisation is not always necessary (Hamilton 2011).

Reproductive Rights, Motives and Decision-making

We have noted the historical justifications for sterilization, in particular the eugenic belief that mental defect was inherited, and the belief that sterilization can have social and therapeutic benefits. More recent research into why women are sterilized, or given long-acting contraception, share common features, and indicate why control of reproduction for women with intellectual disabilities remains a contentious area.

Roets et al. (2006) report their experiences in Belgium in which a young woman with intellectual disabilities and her mother were actively canvassed by professionals to consent to sterilization in ways that appeared disturbingly misleading. While the procedure was first mooted as a means of reducing the discomfort of menstruation, it became apparent that the real concern was the possibility of an unplanned pregnancy (although the woman involved was not in a relationship, nor sexually active at the time). There is also evidence that women in the UK are placed on contraception without making an informed choice when they are neither sexually active nor experience menstrual difficulties that might be resolved by taking the contraceptive pill (McCarthy 2009a). In this study McCarthy found that only five of these women had made a choice to take the contraceptive, the other 18 reported it had been the decision of a parent, carer or GP. Four of the women had started contraception prior to the age of consent (16) and six women were continuing either on the contraceptive pill or on Depo Provera into their mid to late 40s, although not in heterosexual relationships. McCarthy also described the caution inherent in administering contraception to women who were unlikely to become pregnant as the 'just in case approach', a belief that had been internalized by some of the women themselves. The attitude of the majority of her respondents was characterized as 'passive', accepting that others made the decision for them, and that they would be resisted if they sought to make a different choice: 'my dad would have something to say about it' said one (McCarthy 2009a: 367).

So, if women themselves are not making the decision, the question remains: who is? Mothers frequently appeared to instigate sterilization procedures. This was true for Ebba, the self advocate cited above, also for the majority of cases studied by Stansfield, Holland Clare (2007), and evidence from an earlier research study by Patterson–Keels et al. (1994, quoted in Stansfield 2007). In a case cited by Hollomotz (2011), a mother in law worked with the social worker to persuade a young woman with intellectual disabilities to have the operation. Interestingly, this was also true in a qualitative Taiwanese study by Chou and Lu (2011), who highlighted potential similarities in western and non-western approaches. In their small sample of 11 primary carers and four women with mild intellectual disabilities, Chou and Lu reported that mothers in law were significant decision makers, as were husbands. This is explained that because the majority of the women were married and it was customary for their husband's family to take responsibility for decision making.

It is also possible that paid carers are influential, though this is an area that is under-researched. McCarthy (2009a) describes a complex set of relationships between carers, family members and family doctors which influenced the decision to place women on contraceptives. One of the authors (Walmsley), in discussion with a GP, was told that she had resisted expectations from staff at a local residential home to give Depo Provera injections to all the female residents to manage their menstruation. The previous GP who attended the home had performed this routinely.

The reasons given for sterilization in the various studies cited so far have common features. The first is the desire for a permanent solution to potential pregnancy, and concern about who may care for any grandchild. This was cited by Pauline, a woman from the UK who decided to have her daughter sterilized in 1970, at the age of 20. She stated in an interview:

> I mean if she hadn't been sterilized think how many babies she would have had. (Open University on i-Tunes U 2010)

Pauline believed that she was giving her daughter freedom to have sexual relationships without fear of pregnancy – she also assumed that if children were born, then she would have to take care of them. In the study by Chou and Lu (2011) similar considerations applied. The sample included married women with children; it was assumed they were unable to care for them unaided and that to have more would be both onerous to other family members – husbands and mothers in law – and expensive.

However, fear of pregnancy cannot explain the need to sterilize women who are under 24-hour supervision and who have little opportunity to develop relationships with the opposite sex – this was true of the majority of women in the Stansfield, Holland Clare (2007) study. Van Schrojenstein Lantman-de Valk, Rooks and Maaskant (2011) noted that of the 112 women taking contraception in their study, only ten had possible sexual relationships. Like McCarthy (2009a), they also noted the practice of contraception continuing after the menopause or when the likelihood of sexual relationships was limited.

A second significant reason given for sterilizing women is the danger of sexual abuse. In the Taiwanese study one respondent commented:

> My mother was scared that she might be 'chi-fu' (taken advantage of); so she made this decision (tubal ligation)…doing a tubal ligation would make her safe from pregnancy (Chou and Lu 2011: 67-68).

In her interview, Pauline made reference to the occasion when her daughter had been abducted by a man and expressed relief that this had not led to a pregnancy. Sexual abuse, or its consequences, was a feature of the motives for sterilization applications in 25 per cent of the cases considered by Stansfield et al. Sterilization as a response to the possibility of abuse appears to be the result of faulty reasoning. Sterilization, or injected contraception, does not protect against abuse, merely the pregnancy that may result. The consequences can be chilling. For example, John Pring, the journalist who investigated long standing abuse, including rape, at the homes in the Longcare group in Buckinghamshire, England, in the 1990s noted:

> Staff told me disturbing stories including how the GP had given contraceptive injections to at least five of Rowe's female 'favourites' one after the other in a toilet that led off the main reception area, while he continued sitting with Rowe who was sitting at reception (Pring 2005: 4).

The way the General Practitioner (GP) operated, in public, meant that the women had no opportunity to raise with him any objections to the practice, or to tell him of the abuse. This casual practice had enabled the home owner, Gordon Rowe, to continue to rape the women without fear of any consequences. We would suggest that giving contraception to women because they are at risk of sexual abuse is in itself abusive, and points to a lack of regard for their well being.

The final major reason cited for sterilizing women was the management of menstruation, something not mentioned in historical studies. In the Dutch study by van Schrojenstein de Valk et al. (2011) 'problems with menstruation' were cited in 35 cases (57 per cent). These problems included heavy flow, premenstrual syndrome and irregular periods. In a further 24 cases (39 per cent) problems with behaviour related to menstruation were cited, including: mood changes before or during menstruation, crying, self-injurious behavior, obsessive masturbation and problems with maintaining hygiene. Two women in the Chou and Lu (2011) study had hysterectomies to manage menstruation, both at the instigation of their mothers. Another mother in this study mentioned her daughter throwing sanitary towels away. This combined with fear that she would be abused by male students at her day care centre had led them to choose hysterectomy.

Management of menstruation is a task that will not necessarily be welcomed by family members or staff. However, convenience for the carer is a dubious argument for indefinitely placing women on long-acting contraception with possible adverse health consequences. It may explain, however, the practice of administering contraception to women who are – in reality – at very low risk of pregnancy due to age or living circumstances (also noted by McCarthy 2009b, 2010b).

Parenting and Women with Intellectual Disabilities

At several points in this chapter we have suggested that control of women's reproductive capacity is partly to prevent conception, but also to preclude them from rearing children – the historical debates quoted from Somerset in the 1920s make this point very clearly. Of course, struggles for the right to reproduce are experienced by other groups of women who – for moral, political, social and religious reasons – are seen as unfit to mother:

> There is a hierarchy of motherhood with the heterosexual, white, middle-class married woman being the most highly valued. 'Other' mothers, such as the lesbian mother, the mother on welfare, the teen mother and so on, are often stereotyped as inappropriate (Earle and Letherby 2003: 4).

The literature on contemporary parenting by women with intellectual disabilities is far more extensive than that on sterilization, contraception or reproductive rights (see Llewellyn et al. 2010 for a comprehensive international overview). Across the developed world (including Western Europe, Australia and North America), if women with intellectual disabilities get so far as to have children, they are very likely to have them removed. Figures are difficult to come by – partly because the label of intellectual disability is very broad and partly because the label is sometimes applied to people who appear to be 'unfit' parents. However, Llewellyn et al. (2010) quote figures of up to 48 per cent of women having their children removed in Western Europe and Australasia.

Parenting presents one of the most potent challenges to the upholding of women's rights. The literature points to the removal of children based on faulty premises, documented in Australia, Iceland, UK and USA (McConnell et al. 2010). The first assumption is that parental intellectual disability is mistakenly taken for evidence of parental incapacity, and even in some US states is spelt out as a legitimate ground for terminating parental rights. The second is the belief that such people can never become good parents – and that they are subjected to tests and surveillance which other parents might also struggle to surmount, if they had similar treatment (Sigurjonsdóttir and Traustadóttir 2010).

Final Thoughts on Intellectual Disability and Reproductive Futures

It is possible that the sterilization of women with intellectual disabilities is falling into disuse in Western Europe and elsewhere. However, the existing research is limited in its scope, despite the fact that these issues continue to be brought to the public's attention (see McVeigh 2011 for information about a recent Court of Protection case in England). With the advent of Human Rights legislation, the UN Convention on the Rights of Persons with Disabilities to which many western countries are signatories, and in England and Wales, the Mental Capacity Act 2005, things may be changing. It is also possible that the availability of long-acting injectable contraception has made sterilization less attractive, given the legal safeguards surrounding its application. However, as McCarthy points out, ethical, moral and human rights issues have not disappeared just because the technology changes; she argues: 'when a woman .. is put on contraception for most or all of her reproductive life this is arguably a chemical sterilization, yet it has no legal scrutiny' (2010b: 264).

In this chapter, we have laid out the evidence in the published literature on sterilization of women with intellectual disabilities. We have suggested that surgical sterilization is less prevalent than it was in the mid-twentieth century when thousands of women and some men also, were routinely sterilized. In some cases this was technically voluntary, though if the consequences for women were that they remained in institutions if they chose not to accept sterilization, it cannot be seen as a free choice. However, administering contraception to women who are at low risk of pregnancy without their fully-informed consent appears to have continued.

This chapter shows how the reproductive lives of women with intellectual disabilities have been, and continue to be, controlled; and this control has been exercised through a variety of means, both legal and otherwise. We argue that it is imperative that women's agency is recognized, and acknowledge that for some women with intellectual disabilities such practices may create freedom, and may be a positive choice. Indeed, some of the conversations we have had with women indicate that sterilization was an option that they pursued, as it enabled them to participate in sexual relationships free from the worry of getting pregnant (Walmsley 1995).

However, the limited evidence on this subject suggests the wider picture is one of the systematic control of women's lives, creating a series of reproductive losses which have been endorsed and perpetuated by families, carers and practitioners. The practice of 'supervision', for example, means that many people with intellectual disabilities are prevented from expressing themselves sexually. As argued elsewhere,

> Social groups that lack power, also lack the ability to define and regulate their own sexuality. In modern Western societies, sexuality is not seen as an integral part of the lives of disabled people. Disabled people are expected neither to reproduce nor be reproduced (Earle 2001: 435).

Just as supervision controls sexual expression, sterilization – including long-term contraceptive use – prevents a reproductive future.

References

Atkinson, D. and Williams, F. (eds) 1990. *Know Me As I Am: An anthology of prose, poetry and art by people with learning difficulties*. London: Hodder and Stoughton.

Bambrick, M. and Roberts, G.E. 1991. The sterilization of people with a mental handicap: The views of parents. *Journal of Mental Deficiency Research*, 35(4), 353-363.

Board of Control. 1929. *Model Form*. London: Board of Control.

Board of Control. 1926. *Annual Report*. London: Board of Control.

Chou, Y-C. and Lu, Z-Y. 2011. Deciding about sterilisation: perspectives from women with an intellectual disability and their families in Taiwan. *Journal of Intellectual Disability Research*, 55(1), 63–74.

Dyer, C. 1987. Sterilisation of mentally handicapped women. *British Medical Journal*, 294, 825.

Earle, S. 2001. Disability, facilitated sex and the role of the nurse. *Journal of Advanced Nursing*, 36(3), 433-440.

Edgerton, R. 1967. *The Cloak of Competence*. Berkeley: University of California Press.

Engwall, K. 2004. Implications of being diagnosed as a 'feeble-minded woman', in *Gender and Disability Research in the Nordic Countries*, edited by K. Kristiansen and R. Traustadóttir. Sweden: Studentlitteratur, 75-96.

Fennell, P. 1996. *Treatment Without Consent: Law, Psychiatry and the Treatment of Mentally Disordered People Since 1845*. London: Routledge.

Hamilton, C. 2011. New Zealand law on the sterilisation of intellectually disabled women and girls (unpublished report).

Hincks, C.M. 1946. Sterilise the unfit, *Maclean's* (15 February 1946), 19-42.

Hollomotz, A. 2011. *Learning Difficulties and Sexual Vulnerability: A Social Approach*. London: Jessica Kingsley Publishers.

Jackson, M. 2000. *The Borderland of Imbecility: Medicine, society and the fabrication of the feeble mind in late Victorian and Edwardian England.* Manchester: Manchester University Press.

Jones, G. 1986. *Social Hygiene in Twentieth Century Britain*. Worcester: Billing and Sons.

Ladd Taylor, M. 2004. The 'sociological advantages' of Sterilization Fiscal Policies and Feeble Minded Women in Interwar Minnesota, in *Mental Retardation in America*, edited by S. Noll and J. Trent. New York: New York University Press, 281-302.

Laughlin, H. 1926, reprinted 2004. The eugenical sterilization of the feeble-minded, in *Mental Retardation in America*, edited by S. Noll and J. Trent. New York: New York University Press, 225-231.

Llewellyn, G., Traustadóttir, R., McConnell, D. and Sigurjonsdóttir H.B. (eds). 2010. *Parents with Intellectual Disabilities*. West Sussex: Wiley Blackwell.

McCarthy, M. 2009a. Contraception and women with intellectual disabilities. *Journal of Applied Research in Intellectual Disabilities*, 22(4), 363-369.

McCarthy, M. 2009b. 'I have the jab so I can't be blamed for getting pregnant': Contraception and women with learning disabilities. *Women's Studies International Forum*, 32, 198-208.

McCarthy, M. 2010a. Exercising choice and control - women with learning disabilities and contraception. *British Journal of Learning Disabilities*, 38, 293-302.

McCarthy, M. 2010b. The sexual lives of women with learning disabilities, in *Learning Disability: a lifecycle approach*, edited by G. Grant, P. Ramcharan, M. Flynn and M. Richardson. Maidenhead: Open University Press, 259-265.

McConnell, D., Llewellyn, G., Traustadóttir, R. and Sigurjonsdóttir, H.B. 2010. Conclusion: Taking Stock and Looking to the Future, in *Parents with Intellectual Disabilities*, edited by G. Llewellyn, R. Traustadóttir, D. McConnell and H.B. Sigurjonsdóttir. West Sussex: Wiley Blackwell, 241-262.

McVeigh, K. 2011. Mother Drops Legal Bid to Sterilise Daughter with Learning Difficulties. *The Guardian Online* [Online, 20 April]. Available at: http://www.guardian.co.uk/world/2011/apr/20/sterilisation-mental-health-learning difficulties [accessed: 22 July 2011].

Morris, J. (ed) 1996. *Encounters with Strangers: feminism and disability*. London: Women's Press.

Open University on i-Tunes U. 2010. Secret History of Sterilisation. [online] Available at: http://itunes.apple.com/WebObjects/MZStore.woa/wa/viewiTunesUCollection?id=393826122 [accessed: 1 December 2011].

Park, D.C. and Radford, J.P. 1998. From the Case Files: reconstructing a history of involuntary sterilization. *Disability and Society*, 13(3), 317-342.

Patterson-Keels, B.S., Quint, E., Brown, D., Larson, D. and Elkins, T. 1994. Family views on sterilization for their mentally retarded children. *Journal of Reproductive Medicine*, 39(9), 701-706.

Petchesky, R. 1986. Reproductive Freedom: Beyond a Woman's Right to Choose. *Signs* 5: 661-685.

Pring, J. 2005. Why it took so long to expose the abusing regime at Long Care. The Journal of Adult Protection. [Online, June]. Available at: http://findarticles.com/p/articles/mi_qa4124/is_200506/ai_n14801693/pg_6/?tag=content;col1 [accessed: 7 July 2011].

Reilly, P. 1977. *Genetics, Law and Social Policy*. Cambridge, Mass: Harvard University Press.

Roets, G.M., Adams, M. and Van Hove, G. 2006. Challenging the monologue about silent sterilization: implications for self-advocacy. *British Journal of Learning Disabilities*, 34(3), 167-174.

Servais, L., Leach, R., Jacques, D. and Roussaux, J.P. 2004. Sterilisation of intellectually disabled women. *European Psychiatry*, 19(7), 428-432.

Shaw, A. 2004. Attitudes to genetic diagnosis and to the use of medical technologies in pregnancy: Some British Pakistani Perspectives, in *Reproductive Agency, Medicine and the State: Cultural Transformations in Childbearing*, edited by M. Unnithan-Kumar. Oxford: Berghahn Books, pp. 1-24.

Sigurjonsdóttir, H.B. and Traustadóttir R. 2010. Family within a Family, in *Parents with Intellectual Disabilities*, edited by G. Llewellyn, R. Traustadóttir, D. McConnell and H.B. Sigurjonsdóttir. West Sussex: Wiley Blackwell, 49-62.

Stansfield, A. 2007. What factors influence decisions about the sterilization of women with learning disabilities. Unpublished MD, Leeds: University of Leeds School of Medicine.

Stansfield, A., Holland, A.J. and Clare, I. 2007. The sterilization of people with intellectual disabilities in England and Wales in the period 1988-1999. *Journal of Intellectual Disability Research*, 51(8), 569-79.

Stefansdóttir, G. and Hreinsdóttir, E. 2011. It shouldn't be a secret: Sterilisation of women with intellectual disability in Iceland. Nordic Network for Disability Research Conference, Reykjavík, Iceland, 27 May 2011.

TheMentalWeb.com (2011) Legal Resources and Professional Training website. Re F case notes. [Online] http://www.thementalweb.com/index.php/caselaw/cases-pre-2009/93-re-f-mental-patient-sterilisation-1990-2-ac-1-hl.html [accessed: 1 December 2011].

Thomson, M. 1998. *The Problem of Mental Deficiency: Eugenics, Democracy and Social Policy in Britain, c.1870-1959*. Oxford: Clarendon Press.

Tilley, E., Walmsley, J., Earle, S. and Atkinson, D. 2012. 'The Silence is Roaring': Sterilization, reproductive rights and women with intellectual disabilities, *Disability & Society*, 27(3).

van Schrojenstein Lantman-de Valk, H.M.J., Rooks, F. and Maaskant, M.A. 2011. The use of contraception by women with intellectual disabilities. *Journal of Intellectual Disability Research*, 55(4), 434-440.

Walmsley, J. 1995. Gender, Caring and Learning Disability. Unpublished PhD thesis. Milton Keynes: The Open University.

Walmsley, J. and Rolph, S. 2001. The development of community care for people with learning difficulties 1913-1946. *Critical Social Policy*, 21(1), 59-80.

Chapter 3
The Social Shaping of Fertility Loss Due to Cancer Treatment: A Comparative Perspective

Karen Dyer, Khadija Mitu and Cecilia Vindrola-Padros

With more people surviving cancer in developed countries, healthcare providers have begun to pay more attention to cancer patients' and survivors' long-term quality-of-life issues, including the adverse secondary health effects of treatment. One of the most common of these effects is infertility. Certain biomedical treatments for cancer, such as chemotherapy, radiation to the abdominal and pelvic regions, surgery to the reproductive organs, and bone marrow/stem cell transplants, can cause infertility and subfertility in both male and female cancer survivors (Levine et al. 2010). Infertility can be immediate or may occur many years following treatment (Sklar et al. 2006, Stovall and McGee 2010), and a patient's age, type of treatment, and dose received all influence its likelihood (Knopman et al. 2010).

Despite the negative impact of cancer treatment on both male and female fertility, a number of options exist for individuals undergoing cancer treatment to become parents, either biologically or socially. A group of technologies termed *fertility-preservation techniques* has received attention in the last several years; these are technologies that allow men and women to freeze their gametes or tissue prior to the beginning of treatment (Ajala, et al. 2010). Sperm banking and embryo cryopreservation (freezing of fertilized eggs) are routine in developed countries although there is limited access due to cost; other technologies such as ovarian tissue cryopreservation, egg cryopreservation (freezing of unfertilized eggs), and testicular tissue cryopreservation, are still in investigational stages (Fertile Hope 2010). A number of post-treatment parenthood options exist as well, including adoption, surrogacy and the use of donor eggs, embryos, or sperm (Fertile Hope 2010). Most of these fertility-preservation or post-treatment parenthood technologies require the use of artificial insemination (IUI) or in-vitro fertilization (IVF) at a later point when the survivor would like to become a parent, and thus can be quite costly.

The interdisciplinary field of oncofertility has recently emerged in developed countries, such as the United States, United Kingdom, and Australia, with the purpose of addressing the biological and sociocultural aspects of iatrogenic infertility through research and to contribute to the development of policies aimed at the promotion of fertility preservation (Woodruff 2007). Recent studies in this field have demonstrated that cancer patients and survivors often have differential access to needed reproductive technologies. For example, many newly-diagnosed patients are not informed of the risks that cancer treatment poses to their reproductive capacities, let alone receive information about or referrals for fertility-related services from their oncologists (Schover et al. 2002). These discrepancies exist despite the fact that research in developed countries has demonstrated the importance that cancer patients and survivors attach to both fertility and the potential for future parenthood (Schover et al. 2002).

Studies in developing countries are rare; however, some experts in the field of oncofertility have sought to explore how the experiences of cancer-related infertility vary according to the geographical context (Fleetwood and Campo-Engelstein 2010). Scholars have discussed the inequalities produced on the basis of gender, social class, and geographic location in order to highlight the fact that these social categories influence patient diagnosis, cancer treatment, access to fertility-preservation technologies, and fertility outcomes after treatment. Although previous studies represent a notable contribution to understanding the multidimensional character of oncofertility experiences, many of the descriptions provided on what authors call the 'Global South' are based on generalisations and without full examination of the policies and infrastructure of each healthcare system. Furthermore, comparisons between developed and developing countries are also missing.

Accordingly, this chapter will examine how fertility loss and preservation before cancer treatment are shaped in three countries – the United States, Puerto Rico, and Argentina. This chapter uses a comparative analysis of health care policies regarding oncology and infertility treatments to show how biomedical practice and health policies aimed at dealing with the effects of cancer treatment on fertility vary according to the local political-economic context. This analysis is part of ongoing anthropological ethnographic research that is being conducted in these three sites on cancer survivorship and cancer-related infertility, which were selected because they are the authors' research sites. Although these projects are being conducted independently, the authors decided to combine their analysis in this chapter in order to illuminate the diverse range of health strategies these countries employ and the resultant impact upon the availability of ARTs for cancer patients. Specifically, the United States was selected because of its rapidly advancing biomedical technology, particularly in the fields of assisted reproduction and cancer treatment. However, the field of reproductive medicine has been mostly unregulated and access to these services remains restricted to certain groups. Puerto Rico was chosen in order to investigate more deeply the contradiction between the existence of assisted reproductive technology and specialists, with the dramatically restricted access to them that is highlighted by aspects of its colonial relationship with the U.S. Conversely, Argentina is a country in the 'Global South' with limited resources, but which nevertheless has maintained an idea of health as a universal human right and a socialized form of healthcare.

We limit our comparison of these three countries to the public policies, government programs, and the involvement of non-governmental actors focused on patient information and education, and the factors that promote or hinder access to fertility-preservation treatments for oncology patients. We argue that an anthropological, cross-cultural approach to the study of this issue can illuminate the diversity of oncofertility experiences. The organization of the health system is instrumental in understanding how patients obtain cancer treatment, the options available to them for fertility preservation, and, if necessary, the possibility of using ARTs post-treatment. As such, this chapter explores the variability of these three health systems and argues that innovations in treatment do not operate in a social vacuum. Safe and effective technologies exist that allow cancer patients to preserve their fertility prior to treatment; however, access to these technologies, as well as patients' and survivors' experiences of fertility loss in general, is shaped by the organization and ideologies of national health systems, policies, and biomedical practice (Vindrola-Padros et al. 2011). In the three countries discussed below, inequalities exist in terms of access to fertility-preservation techniques, but the *type* of inequality – and the types of barriers limiting patients' access – vary according to the national context.

United States

The U.S. healthcare system is based upon programs provided by both the private and public sectors, although health insurance is largely provided by the private sector (Shi and Singh 2008). While employer-based plans are the major sources of health insurance for people under age 65 (Ward et al. 2008), the public sector also provides insurance through different programs such as Medicaid, Medicare, Children's Health Insurance Program (CHIP), TRICARE, and the Veterans Health Administration. However, many citizens and non-citizens do not qualify for government-provided health insurance, are not provided with health insurance by an employer, or are unable to afford or qualify for private health insurance (Shi and Singh 2008). According to the most recent Census report, approximately 16 per cent of people are uninsured (DeNavas-Walt et al. 2010). The status of insurance coverage affects quality-of-care and treatment outcomes for cancer patients because uninsured adults with cancer are usually diagnosed at more advanced stages of the disease (Halpern et al. 2007; Roetzheim et al. 1999; Ward et al. 2008) and delay seeking care (Virgo et al. 2010).

Lack of healthcare coverage and low socioeconomic status are often cited as factors for existing health disparities between ethnic groups in the U.S. (NCI 2008), while the fragmented healthcare system contributes to a decreased quality-of-care (Taplin and Rodgers 2010). A healthcare reform, known as the Affordable Care Act, was signed into law in 2010, and promises improved and affordable healthcare (Dalton et al. 2010; Virgo et al. 2010). According to the American

Cancer Society, it is anticipated that the new law (to be implemented by 2014) will have a beneficial impact on cancer patients, ensuring that they:

> will no longer a) be denied coverage due to pre-existing conditions, b) be charged more for their coverage because of health status, c) be faced with annual or lifetime coverage limits that cause a sudden termination of care, or d) have to choose between saving their life or their life savings because they lack access to affordable coverage (ACS 2011).

Both cancer treatments and fertility-preservation technologies are advanced and comprehensive in the U.S.; however, various structural issues hinder access to these services. While new technological advancements are ongoing, these technologies remain unaffordable and inaccessible to many cancer patients. Fertility-preservation techniques are very expensive and rarely covered by insurance, adding to the already-existing cost burden of cancer treatment. In addition, social issues such as sexual orientation (Crossley 2006, Rank 2010), ethnicity (Jain 2006, McCarthy-Keith 2010), health status and physical disability (Crossley 2005) can create barriers to accessing fertility-preservation technologies.

Currently, insurance companies in most states do not cover the cost of ARTs. Mandates have been implemented to cover infertility treatment in only 16 states (Quinn et al. 2011); however, discrepancies exist in terms of qualifying for the coverage. Provisions of these laws vary quite significantly between states, and in some cases within states, with respect to defining infertility, mandatory coverage, offering coverage, as well as exclusionary policies regarding coverage of ARTs (Quinn et al. 2011). Although insurance companies generally cover some treatment for iatrogenic conditions related to cancer, such as breast reconstruction after mastectomy and wigs for alopecia, no state currently mandates coverage for *iatrogenic* infertility specifically (Campo-Engelstein 2010). However, new legislation was recently approved in the California Assembly Health Committee that would mandate fertility preservation coverage for cancer patients whose reproductive capacity is threatened by treatment (Charles 2011).

Researchers have documented numerous factors that hinder communication between service providers and cancer patients about infertility as a possible side effect as well as fertility preservation options. The reasons mentioned for *not* discussing or referring cancer patients to reproductive specialists are: a) the perception among providers that fertility-preservation is too expensive for the patient; b) the patient's poor prognosis; c) limited time before cancer treatments; and d) the psychosocial distress the treatment can cause for the patient (Quinn et al. 2009). Researchers have identified a significant gap in the rates of consultation and referral offered by oncologists (Quinn et al. 2009); however, the American Society of Clinical Oncology (ASCO) recently published guidelines recommending that oncologists discuss the possibility of infertility and fertility-preservation options with reproductive-aged patients and offer referrals to appropriate specialists (Lee et al. 2006).

Information about cancer care and treatments, treatment side effects including infertility, and fertility-preservation options are available for patients, service providers and caregivers through a number of governmental and non-governmental organisations (NGO), online networks and support groups. For example, the National Cancer Institute (NCI), the American Society for Clinical Oncology (ASCO), the American Cancer Society (ACS), the American Society for Reproductive Medicine (ASRM), the Society for Assisted Reproductive Technology (SART), Fertile Hope, the Oncofertility Consortium, and the Lance Armstrong Foundation are some of the major organisations that provide information, promote patient advocacy, and build support networks. These organizations and support networks have provided significant space and opportunities for cancer patients and survivors to share their reproductive concerns and problems, interact with others in similar situations, and learn more about options and opportunities that would help them to deal with their own problems and concerns.

Puerto Rico

As an official territory of the United States, Puerto Rico is subject to the federal health laws that govern the 50 states, although the colonial situation that has persisted between the U.S. and Puerto Rico for over 100 years adds a layer of complexity to the analysis of any health situation. For instance, many of the same entitlement programs that operate in the U.S. also apply to Puerto Rico, such as Medicaid – however, the federal contribution is often dramatically lower (Hayashi et al. 2009). For example, the federal matching contribution to Puerto Rico's Medicaid program was $219 million in 2005, versus the $1.7 billion it would have been had the U.S. government used the same calculation it uses for states (Hayashi et al. 2009). A healthcare reform was instituted in 1993 (commonly known as la Reforma), with the goal of expanding health insurance coverage for low-income islanders via Medicaid and thus decreasing disparities in health indicators and access to healthcare (PAHO 2007). At its core was the philosophy of privatization and the '[degovernmentalization] of healthcare, as Government-run health services were considered both inefficient and highly costly for the Government' (PAHO 2007: 8). Prior to the reform, the healthcare system constituted a combination of both private and public resources; however, now medical services have been mostly privatized (PAHO 2007).

While its abiding principle has been to expand access to quality healthcare, a recent evaluation of the reform conducted by the Puerto Rico Department of Health in cooperation with the Pan American Health Organization (PAHO) presented worrisome findings. Although *la Reforma* succeeded in extending health insurance coverage to 93 per cent of the island's population, the quality of care remains poor, the system is fragmented, service rationing has become a problem, prevention systems have been eroded, drug costs have drastically increased, practitioner training has been hampered by the closure of teaching hospitals, patient-doctor relationships have been damaged, and dissatisfaction is high among both patients and providers (PAHO 2007). Further, an evaluation of community health centres in Puerto Rico post-reform revealed that the Medicaid system is chronically and seriously underfunded, with payments that 'cover less than 12 per cent of health centre patient expenditures' (Hayashi et al. 2009: 5). Finally, Puerto Rico ranks lowest on the list of industrialized nations for its health outcomes (PAHO 2007). These findings are incongruous with the fact that it spends the highest proportion of its GNP in the health sector than any other nation in the world (PAHO 2007), illustrating the often-overlooked lesson that health insurance coverage and access to quality healthcare are not one and the same (Hayashi et al. 2009).

Qualitative research with healthcare providers on the island has revealed that even though cancer treatment standards-of-care are established, *la Reforma* does not consistently follow these standards in paying for the full recommended treatment (Simmons et al. 2011). For example, providers report that *la Reforma* will often not pay for necessary tests or for second opinions. In these situations, because residents with the government-sponsored health plan do not have additional insurance, they must choose between getting less than the recommended standard-of-care or pay out-of-pocket.

At the time of writing this chapter, no government policy has addressed insurance coverage of infertility in general or fertility preservation for cancer patients. Relatively few fertility clinics exist on the island; however, most of the clinics in operation offer both fertility-preservation technologies and post-treatment parenthood options. Unfortunately, widespread access to them is restricted by numerous factors. These include high cost; lack of insurance coverage of fertility services – which are often prohibitively expensive, especially in a nation where 50 per cent of residents fall below the federal poverty line (PAHO 2007); geographic location (the clinics are only located in the San Juan metropolitan area, which can be several hours travel time from other parts of the island); limited public awareness of options for fertility preservation; and a combination of cultural, political and economic factors that may limit attention to infertility as a recognised problem (Dyer 2011).

Regarding the latter, for example, since the early 20th Century, the 'official' discourse in the USA surrounding Puerto Rico has been that of overpopulation. The problems that ultimately resulted from industrialization and capitalist expansion, such as the rise of urban poverty and hunger, were blamed on the high fecundity of the poor, non-white residents (Briggs 2002, Lopez 2008). A two-pronged campaign was waged by U.S. and Puerto Rican authorities with the intention of solving the island's 'overpopulation problem': emigration and sterilization (emigration being the temporary 'relief' measure and sterilization/fertility reduction being the long-term solution) (Lopez 2008). Puerto Rico became the site of decades-long experimentation in birth control and a notorious sterilization campaign to reduce the island's population as a way to ostensibly improve its economic condition, and the governmental focus – both Puerto Rican and American – on the overpopulation problem spanned decades (Briggs 2002). However, Briggs has argued that the overpopulation theory is not upheld by the demographic and economic indicators, but rather it has served as a discourse deployed at various moments in time to mask the reality behind the failure of the industrialization program to increase standards of living and decrease poverty – that of colonialist economic policies channelling wealth from the island and into the coffers of American corporations. 'In many ways, overpopulation served as a reply to and encapsulation of this policy concern: something was wrong in Puerto Rico, but it could not entirely be the fault of the United States' (Briggs 2002: 87) – indeed, 'overpopulation' served as a handier and more attractive excuse for the failure of U.S. economic restructuring to bring prosperity to the island's inhabitants and relieve its hunger and poverty.

Regardless of the demographic data, the construction of a nation as overpopulated can have ripple effects that are ultimately reflected in access to health services. In Puerto Rico, it is possible to argue that a socially constructed discourse of overpopulation is connected directly to access and non-access to specific health services – clearly to sterilization and birth control in past decades, and in the present day, to assisted reproductive technologies. The situation in Puerto Rico – whereby few infertility clinics exist and the 'overpopulation problem' has been the overarching discourse throughout much of the 20th century – can be said to reflect a worldwide trend: in countries that have historically been viewed as overpopulated (generally developing countries), infertility and access to ARTs are often treated as a non-issue by scholars, funding agencies and government officials alike (Inhorn 2003). ARTs are neither covered by insurance nor offered through public clinics, and infertility treatment thus become available only for the elites (Inhorn 2003). Tellingly, little research can be located that discusses infertility or ARTs on the island. In essence, the availability of ARTs to cancer patients and survivors (or anybody else) in Puerto Rico reflects larger questions about universal access to assisted reproductive technologies, whether or not access to infertility treatment (and, more broadly, reproduction) is a right or a privilege, and how it applies to contexts in which half of the population falls below the poverty line.

Thus, the history of the overpopulation discourse, birth control movements and sterilization may partially explain the lack of scholarly attention to infertility or ARTs on the island, the non-existent peer-reviewed literature on the fertility loss experiences of individual patients, and limited patient education initiatives. However, incidence rates are increasing for many cancers in Puerto Rico, and mortality rates are declining (Torres-Cintron et al. 2010), creating a situation in which survivorship concerns, including cancer-related infertility, will begin to emerge as priorities.

Argentina

Argentina's healthcare system can be divided in three sectors: private providers, *obras sociales* (a type of union-based social welfare), and public providers (Lloyd-

Sherlock 2005:1895). Since most cancer patients in Argentina access medical treatment in public facilities, we will limit discussion to that area.

In contrast to the ideology that underpins much of the United States and Puerto Rican healthcare system, the Argentine public health system is based on the principle that health is a universal human right that must be ensured by the State. The legal framework that is relevant to the provision of medical services is the Programa Médico Obligatorio (PMO) or Mandatory Medical Program. This program establishes that individuals in need of oncology treatment, antiretroviral therapy, prenatal care, and diabetes, among others, must receive 100 per cent coverage of medical procedures and medication (DIP 2009). In the case of oncology patients without insurance who are accessing services in public hospitals, all services are provided within public health institutions and the drugs necessary for chemotherapy or hormone therapy are provided through the Banco Oncológico de Drogas (Oncology Drug Bank) (Scopinaro and Casak 2002). Oncology patients can also request government assistance in the form of transportation passes, housing subsidies and monthly monetary allocations knows as *pensiones* (Toziano et al. 2004).

In contrast to the problems highlighted by authors who have analysed access to technologies in Latin America (see, for example, Fleetwood and Campo-Engelstein 2010), the case of Argentina raises fewer concerns about treatment affordability due to the implementation of a universalised model of healthcare. This explains why 82 per cent of paediatric oncology patients are guaranteed free medical treatment in public hospitals (INC 2010). This model of healthcare has even transformed the country into a destination for individuals from neighbouring countries who decide to travel to Argentina to access free oncology treatment (Vindrola-Padros 2011).

Equal access to fertility services is promoted nationally through the PMO mentioned above, and on a regional level: for example, legislation exists that guarantees public coverage of fertility-preservation technologies for cancer patients in La Pampa and coverage of two infertility treatments in the Province of Buenos Aires (PLP 2007, 2010).

Cryobank, a sperm bank, was created in 1988 to offer donor sperm and sperm cryopreservation for patients at risk of fertility loss (Osés 2004). Other private institutions provide services for patients dealing with issues of infertility (Raspberry 2007, Sommer 1992) and significant advances have been made in the public sector to make these services widely available (Jofre et al. 2007). The Argentine Society for Reproductive Medicine (Sociedad Argentina de Medicina Reproductiva) has worked with these institutions to promote technological innovation, improve the training of medical professionals, and establish national guidelines for the provision of medical services (SAMER 2005). This organization has also become involved in drafting a proposal for a law regulating the implementation of ARTs.

Even though the Argentine public health system is based on the principle of universal access to healthcare, there are still barriers that limit patients' ability to preserve their fertility prior to treatment and utilise ARTs in the case of infertility.

Several studies have pointed to the challenges faced by oncologists when attempting to provide treatment promptly while taking the necessary measures to protect their patient's fertility (Quinn et al. 2008). This issue, in many ways, cuts geographical boundaries and affects cancer patients in similar ways. However, the structure of the Argentine healthcare system creates additional layers of complexity for both oncologists and patients. Perhaps the most evident factor is the centralization of medical services in the capital of Buenos Aires, leaving a significant portion of the population without medical facilities and trained personnel and forcing patients to leave their place-of-origin to access oncology treatment and ARTs (Scopinaro and Casak 2002, Vindrola-Padros 2011). The disarticulation and lack of communication between hospitals and clinics, the lack of training of medical professionals on the early symptoms of cancer and the scarcity of resources in public hospitals generate delays in diagnosis and treatment and limit the possibility of patients to safeguard their fertility (Scopinaro and Casak 2002, Toziano et al. 2004).

Other limitations in accessing ARTs are associated with the social stigma produced by infertility and its representation as a 'female' problem (Sommer 1992); the fact that many technologies are still in an experimental stage or not available in all institutions; and the influence of the traditional image of the family (heterosexual, with children) on the decisions of policymakers, medical professionals, and NGOs to allow or restrict access to these technologies. Raspberry's (2007) ethnographic research on the use of ARTs in Buenos Aires at the beginning of the 21st Century showed that the insemination of single women was not common practice among medical professionals and was seen by some as going against 'nature'. Other ARTs have received similar representation, affecting the options available for oncology patients dealing with infertility. These beliefs are evident in the legislation that has different definitions of parenthood for men and women and directs the administration of reproductive technologies to a couple and not an individual (Sommer 1992, PLP 2010a).

Another concern raised by Raspberry (2007) is the depiction of infertility as a disease and the consequences of this process on the representation of the bodies of infertile women, the medicalization of their lives, and the authority granted to medical professionals for dealing with this 'pathology'. Without discrediting any of these factors, it is important to note that the construction of infertility as a *disease* has another, less discussed, implication in Argentina: to allow patients to demand full coverage for ARTs. If infertility is publicly recognized as a disease, and the State is held responsible for guaranteeing the health of its citizens, then individuals who cannot afford medical treatment have the right to demand public coverage for ARTs. This is the reason why the recognition of infertility as a disease was not only a process installed at the level of government policies, it was also a movement created from the ground up. For instance, *Infertilidad-arg*, a civil society association, has currently created a web portal to connect people having trouble conceiving a child, provide information, and demand the elaboration of an infertility law (Ylarri 2008).

The oncofertility experiences of patients in Argentina differ from those presented in the other countries discussed in this chapter. An analysis of public policies indicates that instead of dealing with issues of affordability of oncology treatment and ARTs, most patients are concerned with overcoming geographical inequalities in the distribution of medical services and obtaining medical assistance without the delays generated by migration and the lack of hospital resources. Furthermore, the prevalence of a universalized model of healthcare forces researchers concerned with oncofertility issues to look at processes of medicalization in a different way, as the pathological representation of infertility can operate as an empowering tool for patients to demand public coverage for ARTs.

Conclusions

Access to innovations in medical treatments and technology are shaped by a number of factors: the ideologies that underpin the priorities and organization of national health systems, health policies enacted at multiple levels of government, and biomedical practices and actors themselves. The United States, Puerto Rico, and Argentina all exhibit varying levels of inequalities in access to fertility-preservation techniques, but the contours of this inequality are context-specific.

The U.S. exhibits hierarchical access to ARTs, with extremely limited insurance coverage of fertility-preservation techniques (or ARTs more broadly). This has led to a high cost burden on the individual patient who wishes to pursue fertility-preservation, resulting in disparities in the midst of available cutting-edge treatment. In Puerto Rico, similar hierarchies of access persist that are complicated by several factors: a colonialist relationship with the U.S. that is reflected by – for starters – the chronic underfunding of Medicaid in comparison to states, a history of population reduction strategies, and the limited of availability of ARTs on the island itself. Finally, because of Argentina's universal healthcare system, the issues involving access present differently. While patients' ability to *afford* ARTs becomes less of an obstacle in a universal healthcare setting, ability to *physically* access them has become the major issue. The centralisation of medical services in the country's capital requires that a large proportion of the population travel great distances for services. Furthermore, the public assurance of coverage for medical conditions recognized in the legislation has led civil society organizations to demand the medicalization of conditions such as infertility to obtain free treatment.

Local variation in health systems, policies, government programs, and involvement of the non-profit/NGO sector in healthcare has significant implications for how patients' and survivors' experience cancer-related infertility—from receiving information at diagnosis, to support services, to ability to access the ARTs themselves. It is no longer possible to talk about oncofertility issues of the 'global south' as if this region of the world corresponded to a homogenous whole in relation to the north. By acknowledging the diversity of how patient experiences are shaped by health systems, researchers can better inform policies and interventions designed to reduce inequalities in access to medical treatments.

Acknowledgements

Sarah Earle wishes to acknowledge support from the Ponce School of Medicine – Moffitt Cancer Center Partnership (NCI Grant #U56 CA118809), the University of South Florida Dissertation Completion Fellowship program, and the Brocher Foundation. Carol Komaromy would like to acknowledge the support from Rensselaer Polytechnic Institute and PEO Foundation. Linda Layne would like to acknowledge the support provided by CONACYT, the Fulbright-Garcia Robles Grant, the University of South Florida, and AAUW.

References

Ajala, T., Rafi, J., Larsen-Disney, P., Howell, R. 2010. Fertility preservation for cancer patients: A review. *Obstetrics and Gynaecology International*, 2010, 1-9.

American Cancer Society (ACS). 2011. *What Does the Affordable Care Act Mean for People with Cancer?* [Online]. Available at: http://www.cancer.org/InYourArea/Eastern/ AreaHighlights/cancernynj-news-aca-guide, [accessed: 22 May 2011].

Briggs, L. 2002. *Reproducing Empire: Race, Sex, Science, and U.S. Imperialism in Puerto Rico.* Berkeley: University of California Press.

Campo-Engelstein, L. 2010. Consistency in insurance coverage for iatrogenic conditions resulting from cancer treatment including fertility preservation. *Journal of Clinical Oncology*, 28(8), 1284-1286.

Charles, B. 2011. Portantino's bill passes key committee. *Pasadena Star-News*, 4 May.

Crossley, M. 2005. Dimensions of equality in regulating assisted reproductive technologies. *Journal of Gender, Race and Justice*, 9, 273.

Dalton, W., Sullivan, D., Yeatman, T. and Fenstermacher, D. 2010. The 2010 Health Care Reform Act: A potential opportunity to advance cancer research by taking cancer personally. *Clinical Cancer Research*, 16(24), 5987 -5996.

DeNavas-Walt, C., Proctor, B. and Smith, J. 2010. *Income, Poverty, and Health Insurance Coverage in the United States: 2009* U.S. Census Bureau, Current Population Reports [Online] Available at: www.census.gov/prod/2010pubs/p60-238.pdf [accessed: 21 May 2011].

Dirección de Información Parlamentaria (DIP). 2009. *Programa Médico Obligatorio: Legislación Nacional Vigente. Buenos Aires, Argentina: Congreso de la Nación.*

Dyer, K. 2011. Reproduction and parenthood among cancer survivors: The survivorship paradigm in Puerto Rican context. Unpublished manuscript.

Fertile Hope. 2010. *Learn More: Parenthood Options* [Online] Available at: http://www.fertilehope.org/learn-more/cancer-and-fertility-info/parenthood-options.cfm [accessed: 18 December 2010].

Fleetwood, A. and Campo-Engelstein, L. 2010. The impact of infertility: Why ART should be a higher priority for women in the Global South, in *Oncofertility: Ethical, Legal, Social, and Medical Perspectives*, edited by T. Woodruff, L. Zoloth, L. Campo-Engelstein, and S. Rodriguez. Boston: Springer, 237-248.

Halpern, M., Bian, J., Ward, E., Schrag, N., Chen, A. 2007. Insurance status and stage of cancer at diagnosis among women with breast cancer. *Cancer*, 110(2), 403-411.

Hayashi, A., Finnegan, B., Shin, P., Jones, E., Rosenbaum, S. 2009. *Examining the Experiences of Puerto Rico's Community Health Centers Under the Government Health Insurance Plan*. Geiger Gibson/RCHN.

Inhorn, M. 2003. Global infertility and the globalization of new reproductive technologies: Illustrations from Egypt. *Social Science and Medicine*, 56, 1837-1851.

Instituto Nacional de Cáncer (INC). 2010. *Análisis de la Situación de Cáncer en la Argentina* [Online] Available at: http://www.msal.gov.ar/inc/equipos_analisis.asp [accessed: 22 May 2011].

Jain, T. 2006. Socioeconomic and racial disparities among infertility patients seeking care. *Fertility and Sterility*, 85(4), 876-881.

Jofré, F, Peyrallo, C., Baravalle, L., Tauscher, P., Serrallonga, S., Erasmo, L., Olivera, C., Grinberg, C., Molina, R., Verona, M. 2007. Impacto de la infertilidad en el hospital público y sus resultados en el periodo 2000-2005. *Reproducción,* 22(1) Available at: http://revista.samer.org.ar/resumen.php?IdArticulo=408 [accessed: 18 February 2011].

Knopman, J., Papadopoulos, E., Grifo, J., Fino, M., Noyes, N. 2010. Surviving childhood and reproductive-age malignancy: Effects on fertility and future parenthood. *The Lancet*, 11, 490-498.

Lee, S.J. 2006. ASCO recommendations on fertility preservation in cancer patients. *Journal of Clinical Oncology*, 24(18), 2917-2931.

Levine, J., Canada, A., Stern, C. 2010. Fertility preservation in adolescents and young adults with cancer. *Journal of Clinical Oncology*, 28(32), 4831-4841.

Lloyd-Sherlock, P. 2005. Health sector reform in Argentina: A cautionary tale. *Social Science and Medicine*, 60, 1893-1903.

Lopez, I. 2008. *Matters of Choice: Puerto Rican Women's Struggle for Reproductive Freedom.* Brunswick: Rutgers University Press.

McCarthy-Keith, D., Schisterman, E., Robinson, R., O'Leary, K., Lucidi, R., Armstrong, A. 2010. Will decreasing assisted reproduction technology costs improve utilization and outcomes among minority women? *Fertility and Sterility*, 94(7), 2587-2589.

National Cancer Institute 2008. *Cancer Health Disparities* [Online: NCI]. Available at: http://www.cancer.gov/cancertopics/factsheet/cancer-health-disparities/disparities_[accessed: 21 May 2011].

Osés, R. 2004 Funcionamiento de un Banco de Semen en Argentina: 20 años de experiencia en la inseminación con semen de donante. *Reproducción*, 17(1), 23-34.

Pan American Health Organization (PAHO). 2007. *Health Systems Profile Puerto Rico*. PAHO/WHO.

Poder Legislativo Provincial (PLP). 2007. Ley 2342 La Pampa 2007.

Poder Legislativo Provincial (PLP). 2010. Ley 14208 Provincia de Buenos Aires 2010.

Quinn, G.P., Vadaparampil, S.T., Gwede, C.K., Bell-Ellison, B.A. and Albrecht, T.L. 2008. Patient-physician communication barriers regarding fertility preservation among newly diagnosed cancer patients. *Social Science and Medicine*, 66(3), 784-789.

Quinn, G., Vadaparampil, S., Lee, J., Jacobsen, P., Bepler, G., Lancaster, J., Keefe, D., Albrecht, T. 2009. Physician referral for fertility preservation in oncology patients: A national study of practice behaviors. *Journal of Clinical Oncology*, 27(35), 5952 -5957.

Quinn, G.P., Vadaparampil, S.T., McGowan Lowrey, K., Eidson, S., Knapp, C. and Bukulmez, O. 2011. State laws and regulations addressing third-party reimbursement for infertility treatment: implications for cancer survivors. *Fertility and Sterility*, 95(1), 72-78.

Rank, N. 2010. Barriers for access to assisted reproductive technologies by lesbian women. *Houston Journal of Health Law and Policy*, 10(2), 115-146.

Raspberry, K. 2007. Conflicted conceptions: An ethnography of assisted reproduction practices in Argentina. The University of North Carolina at Chapel Hill. Available at: http://proquest.umi.com/pqdlink?Ver=1&Exp=05-20-2016&FMT=7&DID= 1328051771&RQT=309&attempt=1&cfc=1 [accessed: 22 May 2011].

Roetzheim, R., Pal, N., Tennant, C., Voti, L., Ayanian, J., Schwabe, A. and Krischer, J. 1999. Effects of health insurance and race on early detection of cancer. *JNCI*, 91(16), 1409-1415.

SAMER. 2005. Fundamentos del proyecto de ley de SAMER presentado ante la cámara de diputados el 28 de Octubre de 2005. *Reproducción*, 20(2), 24-28.

Schover, L.R., Brey, K., Lichtin, A., Lipshultz, L.I., Jeha, S. 2002. Knowledge and experience regarding cancer, infertility and sperm banking in younger male survivors. *Journal of Clinical Oncology*, 20, 1880-1889.

Scopinaro, M. and Casak, S. 2002. Paediatric oncology in Argentina: Medical and ethical issues. *The Lancet Oncology*, 3, 111-117.

Shi, L. and Singh, D.A. 2008. *Delivering Healthcare in America: A Systems Approach*. Sudbury: Jones and Bartlett.

Simmons, V.N., Litvin, E.B., Gwede, C.K., Vadaparampil, S.T., McIntyre, J., Meade, C.D., Brandon, T.H., Quinn, G.P., Jimenez, J.C., Castro, E. 2011. Initial efforts in community engagement with health care providers: Perceptions of barriers to care for cancer patients in Puerto Rico. *Puerto Rico Health Sciences Journal*, 30(1), 28-34.

Sklar, C.A. et al. 2006. Premature menopause in survivors of childhood cancer: A report from the Childhood Cancer Survivor Study. *Journal of the National Cancer Institute*, 98(13), 890-896.

Sommer, S. 1992. New reproductive technologies: A second report from Argentina. *Issues in Reproductive and Genetic Engineering*, 5(3), 291-295.

Stovall, D.W. and McGee, E.A. 2010. How chemotherapy harms ovarian function: and how to assess your patients' risk and reproductive status. *Sexuality, Reproduction & Menopause*, 8(3), 21-28.

Taplin, S.H. and Rodgers, A.B. 2010. Toward improving the quality of cancer care: Addressing the interfaces of primary and oncology-related subspecialty care. *JNCI Monographs*, 40, 3-10.

Torres-Cintron, M., Perez-Irizarry, J., Figueroa-Valles, N.R., de la Torre-Feliciano, T., Ortiz-Ortiz, K.J., Ortiz, A.P., Soto-Salgado, M., Calo, W.A., Suarez-Perez, E. 2010. Incidence and mortality of the leading cancer types in Puerto Rico: 1987-2004. *Puerto Rico Health Sciences Journal*, 29(3), 317-329.

Toziano, R., Walter, J., Brulc, A., Navia, M., Quintana, S., Flores, A. 2004. Perfil sociodemográfico y de la atención de pacientes oncológicos provenientes de cinco provincias en un hospital de atención terciaria. *Archivos Argentinos de Pediatría*, 102(4), 301-307.

Vindrola Padros, C. 2011. The everyday lives of children with cancer in Argentina: Going beyond the disease and treatment. *Children and Society*. Available at: http://onlinelibrary.wiley.com/doi/10.1111/j.1099-0860.2011.00369.x/abstract [accessed: 22 May 2011].

Vindrola Padros, C., Mitu, K., Dyer, K. 2011. Fertility preservation technologies for oncology patients in the US: A review of the factors involved in patient decision-making. *Technology and Innovation*, 13(4).

Virgo, K.S. et al. 2010. Impact of healthcare reform legislation on uninsured and Medicaid-insured cancer patients. *The Cancer Journal*, 16(6), 577-583.

Ward, E., Halpern, M., Schrag, N., Cokkinides, V., DeSantis, C., Bandi, P., Siegel, R., Stewart, A., Jemal, A. 2008. Association of insurance with cancer care utilization and outcomes. *CA: Cancer Journal for Clinicians*, 58(1), 9-31.

Woodruff, T.K. 2007. The emergence of a new discipline: Oncofertility, in *Oncofertility: Fertility Preservation for Survivors*, edited by T.K. Woodruff and K.A. Snyder. Boston: Springer, 3-11.

Ylarri, P. 2008. Buscan una ley en favor de la vida. *Diario Perfil*, 28 September.

Chapter 4
Reconstructing Childbirth Expectations after Pre-eclampsia

Julie Savage

Findings from in-depth qualitative research into 30 women's experiences of pre-eclampsia in the United Kingdom (Savage 2007) reveals how pregnancy and childbirth expectations are reconstructed after suffering from this common but potentially very serious pregnancy complication. Understanding women's expectations of pregnancy is an important aspect of maternity care, providing an insight into how different women might respond to a situation of emerging problematic symptoms. Furthermore, discerning the possible impact of complications upon women's ideas of pregnancy can inform how they might deal and cope with subsequent pregnancies. The reconstruction of ideas about pregnancy identified in this research was characterized by a centralization of the notion of risk. To deal with this risk women deployed three strategies which I refer to as 'avoidance', 'safety in medical surveillance' and 'self-management'. In this chapter, I argue that understanding the nature of these strategies enables professionals to develop ways of empowering women who enter subsequent pregnancies with an 'at risk' status due to previous complications.

The chapter begins with a summary of the nature of pre-eclampsia. Next I describe the methodology before contextualizing my central argument, that risk – which characterizes women's post-complication pregnancy expectations – is not the result of a movement from normality to risk, but a move from *marginalization* to the *centralization* of risk. I then introduce and illustrate the three strategies identified above before concluding with a consideration of their significance for professional practice.

The Nature of Pre-eclampsia

Pre-eclampsia (also called Pregnancy Induced Hypertension) is an illness unique to pregnancy, defined as new hypertension presenting after 20 weeks with significant protein in the urine (proteinuria) and fluid retention (tissue oedema) (National Institute for Clinical Excellence 2011). The cause is unknown but it is thought to be caused by a problem with the placenta. In the UK the illness affects one in ten pregnancies, making it the most common antenatal complication. One in 100 pregnancies will be affected seriously enough to cause some organ damage (most commonly the kidneys and liver) for affected women as well as growth and other problems for their baby; with 500-600 babies dying each year (Action on Pre-eclampsia 2011). According to Neilson (2011) during 2006-08, 22 women died from eclampsia (defined below) and pre-eclampsia in the UK.

Women with early pre-eclampsia might not present with visible signs although it is detectable through routine screening tests. Visible signs and symptoms include swelling, usually of the hands and feet, vomiting, visual disturbances and pain below the ribs. There are three main characteristics of the condition: hypertension, indicating circulatory problems; protein in the urine and oedema (excessive water retention), both linked to inefficient kidney function.

Eventually, pre-eclampsia can affect all the major body organs and can cause a number of serious complications including eclampsia and HELLP Syndrome (haemolysis, elevated liver enzyme levels and a low platelet count). HELLP Syndrome can cause liver and kidney damage, uncontrollable bleeding and strokes (Action on Pre-eclampsia 2010). Eclampsia is characterized by convulsions, with the potential for cerebral haemorrhaging, and liver and heart necrosis (Roberts and Redman 1993); one in every 50 sufferers of eclampsia dies (Action on Pre-eclampsia 2010). The primary danger of pre-eclampsia to the baby is that, as the placenta ceases to work effectively, oxygen and nutrients becomes restricted resulting in slower growth and possible oxygen starvation. The only cure for pre-eclampsia is to deliver the baby, although in rare cases the condition can persist after delivery. Pre-eclampsia is a major cause of prematurity in babies with all its associated problems.

Research Design

The findings presented in this chapter emerged from doctoral research conducted with thirty women who had experienced pre-eclampsia within five years of participating in the study (Savage 2007). The sample was self-selecting via advertisements in national (UK-based) pregnancy magazines and via the newsletters of interested charities: Action on Pre-eclampsia (APEC) and Bliss. Participants' social class position was categorized according to the UK National Statistics Socio-economic Classification (NS-SEC). Using this classification, the sample was over whelmingly middle class. For example, 15 participants belonged to NS-SEC groups 1-2 and only three belonged to NS-SEC categories 4-7. Twenty-seven participants were white with only one describing herself as Black Caribbean and two as 'White Other'. All were aged over 25 years of age with 11 being over 35.

The participants had varying experiences of pre-eclampsia. Twenty-seven experienced pre-eclampsia in their first pregnancy; three suffered pre-eclampsia for the first time after a previous uncomplicated pregnancy. At the time of the study, 16 of the participants had experienced no further pregnancies; six had further pregnancies with no complications. The remaining eight had subsequent multiple experiences of the illness.

I approached the research with a preference for qualitative forms of enquiry informed by a feminist perspective which conceptualizes women's experiences as inherently valid forms of knowledge (Stanley and Wise 1983). At the time, pre-eclampsia was an under-explored phenomenon within the social sciences. Indeed, the sparse attention paid to reproductive loss, including that which can occur through complications such as pre-eclampsia, continues to be highlighted (Earle et al. 2008). To make participants' experiences visible I chose to privilege their subjectivity based on a conviction that the social world is premised upon people's experiences of it. Furthermore, qualitative forms of investigation allow for the research design to evolve over time (Maykut and Morehouse 1994), which I considered necessary given the exploratory nature of the study. Drawing on this approach, semi-structured interviewing was used as the primary method of data collection. I conducted face-to-face interviews with 18 of the participants. Another five were interviewed on the telephone, guided by the thematic schema of the interview schedule, and solicited written accounts from the remaining seven participants.

Early Ideas about Pregnancy

My research revealed that participants initially perceived pregnancy as normal and natural (see also Chapter 5). The fact that pregnancy is a common occurrence led to the assumption of normality, as did positive images of pregnant embodiment within an ideal social and physical environment. Certainly, in the early stages, participants' expectations were devoid of any sense of serious complications. However, exploring the conditions through which these early expectations might be understood, data revealed that they were constructed through a risk assessment process. That is, most participants had engaged with the possibility of risk – and then discounted it. For example, some of them marginalized information they had initially chosen to access about possible risks for various reasons including a lack of embodied experience of such risks which might otherwise have sensitized them. One participant noted: '(U)nless it's something that affects you, you don't actually pick up on it'. Others considered their risks through engagement with lay referral networks which, when devoid of known complications, led them to conclude that risk was not especially relevant to them. For example, one participant commented that, not having 'heard any horror stories from anybody', she assumed that she would experience a trouble-free pregnancy. Thus, initial ideas about the normalcy of pregnancy arose from a consideration of possible risk, and not a lack of engagement with it.

Changing Ideas about Pregnancy: Pregnancy as Risky

A diagnosis of pre-eclampsia brought *back* the reality of risk to participants' lives. Upon diagnosis, the range of emotional consequences were vast: they experienced grief, fear, a sense of failure, an awareness of being alienated from their baby, clinically diagnosed depression and post-traumatic stress syndrome. All of the participants came to reconceptualize pregnancy in a way which distanced it from notions of normality and naturalness, perceiving it instead as an inherently risky phenomenon. One participant said, 'It has made me realise that it can be dangerous…I didn't think you could die from it or come out with serious health problems'.

Participants with a personalized and highly significant sense of risk in future pregnancies responded differently. I have conceptualized these responses to risk as 'avoidance', 'safety in medical surveillance' and 'safety in self-management', and they are discussed next.

Avoidance

During the interviews, some women spoke about avoiding future pregnancy on the basis that it was now simply too risky. Fears were expressed in terms of their own safety and their responsibility to existing children and other family members. A sense of the uncontrollability of the illness was prominent in their explanations of fear. After assuming that pregnancy was 'a pretty natural thing', one participant experienced a particularly severe consequence of pre-eclampsia: post birth she had two eclamptic fits and it was thought she would suffer brain and kidney damage. She was in intensive care for three days. Pre-eclampsia shattered her notion of pregnancy as being something one could safely enter. She also believed that the medical profession would be able to identify any serious problems. Indeed, as argued elsewhere, the medicalization of pregnancy and childbirth have led to women's assumed dependency upon medicine (Arney 1992) and a belief in its omnipotence (Earle et al. 2007). Whilst alternative discourses in the form of New Midwifery (Campbell and Porter 1997) and Natural Childbirth (Balaska 1992) have been promoted as challenges to medical dominance, their power to do so has been disputed (Brooks and Lomax 1999, Annandale and Clarke 1996 respectively). The 'illusion of [medicine's] omnipotence' over pregnancy continues (Earle et al. 2007) and when this cannot be sustained there are consequences for any belief in reproductive control. One participant's good health status did not prevent the illness, and routine surveillance had not predicted the serious complication of her pregnancy. She expressed her fear of suffering again from the disease and, at the time of the research, no longer wanted any more children:

> It's only afterwards … you think … anything could go wrong, so in that way I was lucky to have a healthy child … It has certainly made me think twice about

> any more children … I think the medical side is the main reason for me not wanting any more children.

The perceived lack of visibility of the disease to medical surveillance also resulted in avoidance strategies for some. One participant described pregnancy as something characterized by many positive things which can suddenly be taken away:

> [You are] … looking forward to conceiving and showing you're happy about this pregnancy and this baby growing inside you and then suddenly it can all be taken away in a flash … you know I thought maybe like mothers can die in childbirth a few years back but not in this day and age. You think everything is going to be straightforward … but that's just not the case … we will not risk it again.

Two conditions were identified which reduced the likelihood of participants pursuing an avoidance strategy. First, if there was a belief that the earlier illness had been well controlled with a good outcome for mother and baby, for example: 'Well we felt because we had been through it and [daughter] came on so well … so we decided we would take a chance … otherwise you would never do it again would you …' Second, a belief that pre-eclampsia could not occur again also made adoption of an avoidance strategy less likely, as another participant recounted:

> I went to the doctor and said I was thinking about another pregnancy … he said [he] didn't think it would happen again [that] it doesn't usually … She went through all the risk criteria and basically [said] you have one already so it won't happen again …

So, participants were likely to avoid future pregnancy after pre-eclampsia when their belief in the omnipotence of medicine had been shaken. This avoidance was mediated by medical assurances that it 'wouldn't happen again', as well as by positive pregnancy outcomes which showed that it could all end happily.

Safety in medical surveillance

For participants who considered pregnancy to be risky, submitting to medical surveillance and supervision was a strategy they used to cope with another pregnancy; and, increased consultations with health professionals were positively embraced. In thinking about a future pregnancy, one participant commented: '[A] lthough I am anxious about a future pregnancy, my husband and I feel it is worth proceeding. I visited my consultant who assured me…that I could have more frequent antenatal appointments.' Knowing her risk of experiencing pre-eclampsia again, another participant described how her awareness of increased supervision mitigated her fear of becoming pregnant again: 'I know there is a chance that I could have the same problems again but I also know that my GP will keep an extra eye on me next time.'

The strategy of medical surveillance was further illustrated by participants who become pregnant again. One had been cynical about the necessity of hospital stays in her first pregnancy. After developing her understanding of the dangers of the disease and centralizing this risk, her second pregnancy was characterized by a resignation to surveillance and increased intervention: 'The second time round I knew about it and I was happy to do whatever I was told to do.'

Defining pregnancy as risky also led some participants to reconsider their ideas on hospitalized births. For example, one participant had previously considered a home birth as 'romantic' and had wanted such an experience. Entering her second pregnancy after experiencing pre-eclampsia in the first, she had no intention of having a birth without direct medical supervision and intervention which would take the form of a planned caesarian, she said: 'I do not want the risk of anything else going wrong … I want to sort out the date and get him or her out.'

In these accounts, experiential knowledge was used to embrace, or at least accept medical surveillance and intervention during pregnancy to ameliorate the risks of potential complications from the risk of pre-eclampsia.

Self-management

The third strategy used by participants to deal with a reconceptualization of pregnancy as risky was to take control of it themselves. Though this response to risk is given separate consideration here, in their lived experiences it was sometimes intertwined with the previous response of submission to medical expertise insofar as this 'taking control' was, in some cases, informed by dominant medical discourses on pre-eclampsia.

Some women attempted to monitor and reduce risk through lifestyle changes. Factors identified as risky by participants when they described their early perceptions of pregnancy included working, going on holiday, not eating correctly, becoming stressed and carrying heavy objects. Whilst this is seen most clearly in the accounts of those who entered a further pregnancy, it is also visible amongst those who were at the stage of only contemplating the possibility of further children. The perceived need to reduce risk through lifestyle changes is shown in one participant's reflections: 'I have lost six and a half stone and I will lose another couple, just to basically help the chances, although weight has nothing to do with it …' Another shared: 'I learnt from my first pregnancy that you don't go out to work; you don't rush around the house. You don't push yourself. You keep yourself at a steady pace and what doesn't get done, well tough.'

A further aspect of self-management to control or reduce the risk of pregnancy involved developing expertise about pre-eclampsia. This expertise involved a medically-defined understanding of pre-eclampsia, its detection and means of control. Participants seeking such information accessed it via the internet, books and support groups like Action on Pre-eclampsia. This allowed some to develop a sense of control. Thinking about the possibility of having another baby, and already in possession of medical knowledge, one participant explained:

> … [T]hat's why I contacted APEC and I do think it's important … I actually needed the knowledge. I needed to know everything, to reassure me that I had not done anything wrong and that also if I do ever get through another pregnancy that I know all the facts … and I (would) be more in control. I can say well this is what I have had before and you know this is what I want; you know to keep an eye on it I suppose.

This developing expertise was sought and changed their subsequent experience. All participants reported a 'better' experience because they felt more in control. After a first experience of pre-eclampsia, one participant had concluded that hospital was the safest place to control the risk associated with her second pregnancy and birth. However, she ' … no longer trusted' the professionals after believing that her baby should have been delivered earlier than it was. From this experience she was willing to challenge them on the basis of her developed understanding:

> I knew what to ask then as well. I knew what the questions were. I knew what it meant if I had a plus of protein in my urine. I didn't know what it meant the first time … [in the second pregnancy] … I wouldn't have accepted what they'd told me. You know 'ok it's only a trace'. I wouldn't have stood for that. I also know for a fact a couple of times going and not having my urine checked…I remember going down to the doctors. I didn't have a sample bottle. I remember the nurse saying to me, do you have a sample? I said, no I do not and she said well make sure you bring it next time. At that time I thought oh well, it's fine … and that stuck in my mind … but yes the second time around I made sure it was tested because I knew.

Another participant's developing expertise gave her the confidence to become greatly involved in the monitoring of her own condition through having urine sticks to test for proteinuria and taking her own blood pressure:

> I probably also knew a lot more and felt much more in control and I did things like if my blood pressure went up I would take a twenty four hour urine test … I would take it right away to clinic, that saved a bit of time being admitted … my main aim was to stay out of hospital (for as long as possible) and I did …

Participants' medical expertise developed both through the information they accessed and through drawing on their experiential knowledge. For example, one described how she had developed expertise based on her embodied previous experience and subsequent reading which enabled her to take some control and be more assertive in asking about the nature of medical surveillance.

> They were telling me things and I was saying but that's not right, so I was actually telling them … I would go into the unit and have my blood pressure measured and I would watch them, I would be watching for every reaction … I would be like what's the number and they would say one hundred and five and I would say so when am I going downstairs … what's the reading of the protein in the urine, well's there's a little bit of protein, well what's the reading, is it one, two or three plusses …

All of the study participants who chose to self-manage the risks associated with pre-eclampsia drew on medical knowledge and expertise. They used this newly developed expertise to take control of their experiences but instead of 'submitting' to medical surveillance, used this strategy to inform themselves, often becoming active participants in their (self) care, and sometimes challenging medical expertise.

The Professional Implications of Women's Changed Understanding of Risk

I began this chapter by asserting the importance of understanding women's pregnancy expectations. Discerning these expectations may help to identify women's possible responses to emerging problems. Understanding the impact of pregnancy complications upon women's ideas of pregnancy allows professionals to identify the possible range of responses should these ideas shift from the marginalization of risk to its centralization.

Changing Childbirth, the report of the Expert Maternity group, published in 1993 was considered a radical departure from previous maternity reports since it claimed to promote a woman-centred approach to the organization of maternity services. The report asserted the need for services to make full use of midwifery skills in the context of uncomplicated pregnancies. Whilst the report *Safer Childbirth* (2007: 1) acknowledged the role of midwives as, 'partners with obstetricians, anesthetists and pediatricians, in the care of women with complex and complicated labours', midwifery continues to define itself primarily in relation to normal pregnancies. For example, the Royal College of Midwives' *Midwifery Practice Guideline* (2008) explicitly excludes women with complications, instead briefly identifying the expectation that where there is concern, referral to an obstetrician should take place. Their *Position Paper on Normal Birth* (2005) makes it clear that the skill of the midwife resides in the supporting and maximisation of normal birth. I have suggested elsewhere (Savage 2007) that women with complications also require and indeed seek the care ordinarily associated with that provided by midwives. The strategies adopted by women to deal with a situation whereby any future pregnancy becomes considered risky reveal opportunities for midwives to support women when pregnancy is defined as 'at risk', whether that risk is realized or not.

Managing assumptions regarding risk

This chapter illustrates how some participants chose to avoid future pregnancy because their heightened sense of risk led them to conclude that safety could only be assured through an avoidance strategy. The seeming uncontrollability and invisibility of pre-eclampsia were two main features of their reflections. Neilson (2011) identified that of the 22 women in the UK who died from pre-eclampsia and eclampsia in the years 2006-08, 20 were associated with substandard care provided within both hospitals and the community. This suggests that negative outcomes, in this case mortality, are *not* an inevitable outcome of the disease *per se*, but rather a result of substandard care. If women are to choose to avoid future pregnancy it should be on the basis of a thorough understanding of their particular risk rather than on heightened fear emerging from the assumption of its uncontrollability.

Whilst early on in the disease pre-eclampsia can be symptom-less, and thereby 'invisible' to the woman herself, there *are* clinical indicators which can be identified through ante-natal screening. Women who have experienced complications need to be supported in identifying and understanding information about the possibility of effective management of future risk. A consistent theme that emerged from participants' reflections was the experienced restrictions on information concerning pre-eclampsia; this was identified as an area for improvement. One participant felt that:

> They could have told me about it beforehand ... [T]hen when you come down for your antenatal and you are going to come and offer your arm and your little pot of wee, there is some information on it ... I am fairly confident that in those three days when I was thinking I've not peed as much as I should, I would have been thinking I wonder if this is a sign of pre-eclampsia and would have gone to the GP.

As noted earlier, avoidance was less likely to be adopted by participants if their previous experience of pre-eclampsia had been well controlled. Such control would be likened with early detection and intensive management. Whilst midwifery distances itself from pregnancy which cannot be defined as 'normal', in the UK the pre-eclampsia community guideline (PRECOG) details an evidence-based risk assessment plan for the community and identifies that when such plans are constructed women's emotional and midwifery needs *should* be accounted for (Milne 2005). My research demonstrated the importance of recognizing and acting upon such needs. Within a situation of intense medical surveillance due to complications, whilst many of the participants expressed gratitude for the technological expertise, five explicitly identified a failure to recognize their holistic needs. For example, one commented that whilst the medical care was very good '...it was very impersonal and very uninformative.' Another remembered how she was simply 'treated like a person in a bed.' There is a relationship between being informed and experiencing intensive health care more positively. For one participant reflecting upon her experience of needing to have her baby delivered at 34 weeks, the ability of the midwife to communicate to her both clearly and sensitively transformed her experience: '…the fear departed because you actually felt in control of what was going on. I think it is the lack of control that is the scary bit, not knowing exactly what is happening…'

In describing the avoidance response earlier, this chapter identified another factor which would reduce the likelihood of the strategy being adopted: the belief that pre-eclampsia would not reoccur. Such a belief can never be fully informed since evidence demonstrates that women who have experienced pre-eclampsia are at risk again and should be categorized as such (National Institute for Clinical Excellence 2003). Therefore, just as avoidance based on a lack of information is dis-empowering to women, so too is an assumption of future pregnancy normality after pre-eclampsia. Midwifery practice is therefore of great significance within a context of possible and actual risk and necessary high levels of surveillance and intervention as the profession informs and supports women during and post pregnancy complications and as women consider their future at-risk status.

Empowering Women through Surveillance

Submission to medical expertise provides some women with a strategy to deal with the centralization of risk. Consequently, women may come to define good care in terms of the intensity of medical supervision. For example, one participant commented:

> I saw my midwife when I was four weeks and three days pregnant and was put onto low dose aspirin. I took these until thirty-four weeks. All through the pregnancy my care was excellent. I never went longer than two weeks without seeing anyone, usually the community midwife one week, the hospital consultant the next. I had regular scans to check the baby was growing okay …

However, this should not be conflated with an acceptance of a system of care which fails to recognize the holistic needs of women. Whilst, as illustrated previously, women may come to define 'good care' as high levels of intervention, these were considered necessary, not just for clinical medical surveillance, but for supporting women psychologically as they experienced what they had come to consider risky. When fear emerges, the role of the midwife in providing reassurance is important. For example, one participant shared that:

> Several times I got myself into a bit of lather, convinced it was all happening again and each time I phoned my midwife and she would be with me within a hour, never complaining about paranoid me, just ready to reassure me.

The framework for ensuring a woman-centred approach to care which recognizes the needs of women beyond issues of mortality and morbidity need not be sacrificed in situations where pregnancy risk is dominant. My data showed how women experiencing pregnancy complications can find themselves in a situation of obstetric intervention which marginalizes their holistic needs. Women's reconceptualization of pregnancy as risky and their subsequent dependency upon medical interventions is precisely the situation where the skills of midwifery can be used. The key principle of midwifery care is to provide good information and to empower women to be involved in decisions about their own pregnancy (Royal College of Midwives 2008). Submission to obstetric care does not have to be passive – rather, through providing support and information, the midwife may be best placed to empower women to actively participate in this management of risk. The third strategy of self-management developed by women who come to centralize risk might give some insight into the practical expression of this.

Supporting Self-management

Participants who adopted self-management to manage their perception of pregnancy as inherently risky sought to take of control of the risk through life-style changes and developing expertise. This focus upon understanding tended to emerge in situations where a woman's previous experience of pre-eclampsia made evident her lack of understanding:

> To be honest I thought the swelling … people get swollen ankles when they get pregnant … [T]he epigastric pain was … I remember being quite pleased about it because I read in my book that you might get some pain because your ribs move a bit, because your uterus is pushing up. I remember that 'cos I was pleased with the pain 'cos it must have meant that I was getting bigger …

Self-management strategies require accurate information. The role of the midwife in relating evidence-based life-style risks and broader knowledge regarding pre-eclampsia is essential if women's self-management in this area is to be effective. Information about pre-eclampsia should be available to all pregnant women with its commonality and symptoms emphasized. Post pre-eclampsia it is clear that they should be offered support in identifying further information should they want it. Routine ante-natal testing is a vital means of detecting the disease even before signs and symptoms become evident. Some participants dealt with the centrality of risk by proactively ensuring that appropriate ante-natal checks were carried out. I argue that midwives should positively encourage women to mount a challenge where ante-natal testing is not administered appropriately. Furthermore, midwives should consider the benefits that women might derive from being carefully advized about and then supported in conducting regular self-testing of urine and blood pressure.

Conclusions

In their early expectations of pregnancy many of the study participants had marginalized the possibility of high levels of medical surveillance and intervention. This emerged as a consequence of considering the various dimensions of risk as they pertained to their pregnancy but then largely discounting them. However, the experience of pre-eclampsia led to a reconceptualization of risk and in this chapter I have identified and illustrated three responses to this reconceptualization. Whereas for some it led to an avoidance of pregnancy, for others it led to a belief that submission to medical surveillance was of central importance in defining their future pregnancy. However, some participants, sought to control their perceived pregnancy risks through a process of self-management. I have suggested some possible implications of these strategies at the level of professional practice.

If the role of midwife is to be 'with woman' then the profession should be encouraged to engage even more with pregnancies defined as potentially abnormal. The central skills of the midwife in supporting and informing women so that their care indeed may be woman-centred can be in many ways transpose into situations of necessary obstetric supervision and surveillance. Here, I suggest that each strategy adopted bring opportunities for midwives to do what they do best: to inform, support and empower women.

References

Action on Pre-eclampsia. 2010. *Pre-eclampsia: The Basics*. [Online]. Available at: http://www.apec.org.uk/preeclampsiabasics.htm [accessed: 25 May 2011].

Annandale, E. and Clarke, J. 1996. What is gender? Feminist theory and the sociology of human reproduction. *Sociology of Health and Illness*, 18(1), 17-44.

Balaskas, J. 1992. *Active Birth: The New Approach to Giving Birth Naturally.* Boston: Harvard Common Press.

Brooks, F. and Lomax, H. 1999. Labouring bodies: mothers and maternity policy, in *Social Policy and the Body: Transitions in Corporeal Discourses*, edited by K. Ellis and H. Dean. London: Macmillan Press.

Campbell, R. and Porter, S. 1997. Feminist theory and the sociology of childbirth: a response to Ellen Annandale and Judith Clarke, *Sociology of Health and Illness*, 19(3), 348-358.

Centre for Maternal and Child Enquiries (CMACE). 2011. Saving Mothers' Lives: Reviewing Maternal Deaths to make Motherhood Safer: 2006–08. The Eighth Report on Confidential Enquiries into Maternal Deaths in the United Kingdom. *BJOG*. 118(Suppl. 1).

Department of Health. 1993. *Changing Childbirth: The Report of the Expert Maternity Group*. London: HMSO.

Earle, S., Komaromy, C., Foley, P. and Lloyd, C.E. 2007. The social dimensions of reproductive loss. *Practising Midwife*, 10(6), 28–34.

Earle, S., Foley, P., Komaromy, C. and Lloyd, C.E. 2008. Conceptualizing reproductive loss: A social sciences perspective. *Human Fertility*, 11(4), 259–262.

Lewis, G. 2011. 'The women who died', in Centre for Maternal and Child Enquiries (CMACE). *Saving Mothers' Lives: Reviewing Maternal Deaths to make Motherhood Safer*: 2006–08. The Eighth Report on Confidential Enquiries into Maternal Deaths in the United Kingdom. *BJOG*, 118(Suppl.1).

Maykut, P. and Morehouse, R. 1994. *Beginning Qualitative Research: A Philosophic and Practical Guide.* London: Routledge/Falmer.

Milne, F. 2005. The Pre-eclampsia Community Guideline (PRECOG): How to Screen for and Detect Onset of Pre-eclampsia in the Community. *British Medical Journal*, Mar 12, 330(7491): 576-580.

National Institute for Clinical Excellence. 2003. *Antenatal care: Routine care for the healthy pregnant woman*. [Online]. Available at: http://www.nice.org.uk/nicemedia/pdf/CG6_ANC_NICEguideline.pdf [accessed: 15 April 2011].

National Institute for Clinical Excellence. 2011. *Hypertension in pregnancy: the management of hypertensive disorders during pregnancy*. London: Royal College of Obstetricians and Gynaecologists Press.

Neilson, J. 2011. Pre-eclampsia and eclampsia, in Centre for Maternal and Child Enquiries (CMACE). Saving Mothers' Lives: reviewing maternal deaths to make motherhood safer: 2006–08. The Eighth Report on Confidential Enquiries into Maternal Deaths in the United Kingdom. *BJOG*, 118 (Suppl. 1).

Office for National Statistics 2000. *Introduction: the National Statistics Socio economic Classification*. [Online]. Available from: http://www.ons.gov.uk/ons/guidemethod/classifications/archived-standard-classifications/ns-sec/index.html [accessed: 25 November 2010].

Roberts, J.M. and Redman, C.W. 1993. Pre-eclampsia: more than pregnancy induced hypertension. *Lancet*, 342(8869), 504.

Royal College of Midwives. 2005. *Definition and the RCM Position Paper*. [Online]. Available from: http://www.rcmnormalbirth.net/default.asp?sID=1103625596157 [accessed: 1st May 2011].

Royal College of Midwives. 2008. *Midwifery Practice Guideline: Introduction*. [Online]. Available at: http://www.rcm.org.uk/college/policypractice/guidelines/practice-guidelines [accessed: 11 July 2011].

Royal College of Anaesthetists, Royal College of Midwives, Royal College of Obstetricians and Gynaecologists, Royal College of Paediatrics and Child Health. 2007.

Safer Childbirth: Minimum Standards for the Organisation and delivery of Care in Labour. London: Royal College of Obstetricians and Gynaecologists Press.

Savage, J. 2007. *The Experience of Pre-eclampsia: Developing the Feminist Critique of Medicalized Childbirth*. Unpublished PhD. Milton Keynes: The Open University.

Stanley, L and Wise, S. 1983. *Breaking out: Feminist Consciousness and Feminist Research.* London: Routledge and Kegan Paul.

Chapter 5

Diabetes and the Pregnancy Paradox: The Loss of Expectations and Reproductive Futures

Sarah Earle and Cathy E. Lloyd

In modern western societies, pregnancy, childbirth and early motherhood are often understood, and experienced, paradoxically. On the one hand, these experiences are epitomized as the most natural, joyous, special and even empowering of experiences. On the other, they can also be experienced as some of the most medicalized, technocratic, traumatizing and disempowering of times. In this chapter we argue that diabetes in pregnancy sits at the very intersection of this paradox.

In 1989 the St Vincent's Declaration *Diabetes Mellitus in Europe* called for the outcome of pregnancies in women with pre-existing (Type 1) diabetes to be comparable with those of women without this condition; this declaration was made under the aegis of WHO Regional Office for Europe and the International Diabetes Federation. However, over 20 years on, diabetes remains the most common medical complication in pregnancy and is associated with increased risks to life and health for mother and baby including, obstetric complications, increased rates of caesarean delivery, increases in congenital abnormalities and perinatal mortality and morbidity (CEMACH 2007). Drawing on the relatively limited social sciences literature on this topic and on the findings of a consultation process involving women with pre-existing (Type 1 and Type 2) and gestational diabetes in pregnancy in the UK, this chapter sets out to explore how through this paradox, women with diabetes can experience a sense of reproductive loss throughout the pregnancy process.

Diabetes in Pregnancy: What are the Risks to Health?

Rates of diabetes during pregnancy are rapidly increasing in the UK, and elsewhere, and are seen to be a serious public health concern (CEMACH 2007). These increased rates are mainly due to the rapid rise in the numbers of women who have Type 2 diabetes and it has been suggested that this is associated with an increased prevalence of British people who are overweight and obese (Coulthard et al. 2008). Type 2 diabetes typically occurs later in life, and is usually treated with diet and increased physical activity initially but medication and/or insulin injections are often required to control the condition. Type 1 diabetes begins during childhood or early adulthood and requires the use of multiple daily insulin injections and testing of blood sugar levels in order to maintain health and wellbeing for the rest of one's life.

Outcomes for women with all types of diabetes during pregnancy tend to be measured in terms of infant morbidity such as congenital abnormalities, and infant and maternal mortality. A key report from the Confidential Enquiry into Maternal and Child Health, which focused on women with pre-existing Type 1 diabetes, highlighted a five-fold increase in still-births, a three-fold increased risk of perinatal mortality and a two-fold increased risk of congenital abnormalities (CEMACH 2010). The same report highlighted that preterm delivery rates were more than five times more common in women with Type 1 diabetes compared to women without this condition, and caesarean section rates were nearly trebled.

Research suggests that women who develop gestational diabetes (GDM) also have an increased risk of morbidity and mortality. GDM – diabetes which appears during pregnancy and usually disappears postnatally – occurs when the body cannot produce enough insulin to meet the extra needs of pregnancy. It is associated with being overweight and also with a family history of Type 2 diabetes and is therefore also increasing in frequency as both of these conditions become more common. Although it usually goes away after childbirth, women with GDM have an increased risk of developing Type 2 diabetes later on in life as well as having GDM in subsequent pregnancies. Barahona and colleagues (2005) noted that gestational diabetes was a predictor for adverse maternal outcomes including hypertension, and adverse neonatal outcomes including prematurity, low Apgar scores, and perinatal mortality. However, adverse outcomes are more significant for women with pre-existing diabetes compared to women who develop diabetes in pregnancy. Both Type 2 diabetes and GDM are more common in women from minority ethnic groups and those living in deprivation (Casson 2006).

During pregnancy and childbirth, all types of diabetes introduce a range of challenges for women and those providing their care. Having diabetes means incorporating a whole range of self-care behaviours into daily life including blood testing, medication taking, and dietary restrictions. People with diabetes are also more likely to have mental health problems such as depression in comparison to people without this condition (Lloyd et al. 2010).

Current UK recommendations for the care of women with diabetes before and during pregnancy focus on medical considerations, especially achieving good blood glucose control. The main aim of this care is to reduce the risk of complications during pregnancy and childbirth. However, women have other non-clinical needs such as the need for peer and/or social support that are not always addressed, and which can affect the experience of pregnancy and childbirth.

Consulting with Women about their Experiences

Research in the UK has focused predominantly on the clinical care of women with diabetes in pregnancy, with little attention paid to women's psychosocial needs, experiences and expectations of care, in spite of the National Institute for Health and Clinical Excellence (NICE 2008) guidelines which recommend that women's needs and preferences for care should be taken into account. To address the relative lack of research in this area, a multidisciplinary team of academic researchers and health professionals worked together to prepare a proposal to be submitted to the UK National Institute of Health Research (NIHR) *Research for Patient Benefit* Programme.

Women with diabetes who had recently had a baby at a large NHS Trust in the West Midlands, UK, were invited to attend one of four discussion groups as part of a consultation process. The purpose of the discussion was to explore experiences of diabetes in pregnancy as a means of identifying significant potential research themes. Seventeen women of white Caucasian (n=13) or South Asian Mirpuri (n=4) origin participated in the discussions which were facilitated by either one or two academic members of the multi-professional group and attended by the specialist diabetes midwife, who was also a member of that group. The discussions, each of which lasted approximately 90 minutes, were digitally recorded and transcribed *verbatim*. The groups were held in an informal setting and the majority of women who attended brought their babies and/or younger children. Some of the data generated via this consultation process are presented here, together with data drawn from other social sciences literature in the field.

Reproductive Loss and the Loss of Futures and Expectations

As we have highlighted elsewhere, the study of human reproduction often focuses on reproductive success, and on the struggles to achieve this (Earle et al. 2008). The discourses that surround the subject of pregnancy and childbirth usually focus on positive outcomes and happy endings, without always acknowledging experiences of loss, many of which are incredibly common. Layne (2003) suggests that such discourses merely serve to exacerbate the experiences of those whose pregnancies do not end happily or; indeed; where pregnancies do not occur at all. As argued previously, reproductive loss refers to a wide range of experiences, including early and late miscarriages, stillbirth, perinatal, infant and maternal death, as well as infertility and assisted reproduction (Earle et al. 2008). To extend this even further, we argue here that diabetes in pregnancy, where pregnancies come to be defined as high risk, and mothers and children as at-risk, can also be included within the broad umbrella of reproductive loss. That is, in the widest sense, reproductive loss refers to the loss of expectations *vis-à-vis* idealized notions of 'normal', 'natural' and trouble-free pregnancies.

Previous research indicates that women who experience diabetes in pregnancy are often subject to additional surveillance. For example, a Swedish study of midwives revealed their beliefs that mothers-to-be with diabetes had a moral obligation towards their foetus to make healthy choices (Persson et al. 2010). This obligation manifested itself as an increased monitoring and control of the pregnancy by the midwife. The midwives in this study also admitted to monitoring and questioning any behaviour that deviated from, or was found to contradict, their prescribed advice. When 'non-compliance' with their advice occurred, this was regarded as irresponsible behaviour by the pregnant woman and often caused friction in the care relationship. Other research has considered the situation from the point of view of pregnant women. One such study (Evans and O'Brien 2005) argues that women who have diabetes in pregnancy describe it as 'living a controlled pregnancy'. In other words, juggling diabetes and pregnancy was found to limit women's ability to be autonomous, limited their control of normal daily activities and subjected them to day-to-day control and supervision by both internal and external forces; that is, women could be subjected to self-surveillance and surveillance by health professionals and even others. Such women characterize their pregnancies as a series of personal struggles to balance their desire for autonomy with the challenges of being under constant surveillance and adapting to required lifestyle changes. Of course, managing diabetes can be a frustrating and challenging experience whatever the circumstances. Living with diabetes has been described elsewhere as an 'ever-present moral dilemma' whereby individuals try to integrate their condition and their prescribed regime within their desired lifestyles (Watts, O'Hara and Twigg 2010). This moral dilemma may well be compounded when combined with the moral expectations placed upon and internalized by pregnant women. Not only do such women need to factor in what it means to be a 'good' or 'successful' person with diabetes but, also, a 'good' mother-to-be with diabetes.

The following part of this chapter draws on the data from the discussion groups to examine women's experiences of pregnancy and diabetes, focusing on care during pregnancy, childbirth and the immediate post-natal period.

Women's Experiences of Diabetes and the Pregnancy Process

Care during Pregnancy

Our discussions highlight how care during pregnancy seems to be dominated by medical surveillance and a focus on *diabetes* care, rather than on pregnancy, to the detriment of an anticipated 'normal', ante-natal experience. As one respondent succinctly summarises:

> … as time went on I just accepted that … it was more about the diabetes than the pregnancy.

However data show that there were high expectations of service provision although this was often reported as unfulfilled in practice. As highlighted by previous studies (Persson et al. 2010, Evans and O'Brien 2005) the over-riding focus on diabetes care – rather than the experience of being pregnant – led to some dissatisfaction even if the clinical (diabetes) care was perceived as good quality. Two participants commented:

> … the diabetes side was fantastic, but may be just a bit more support with just being pregnant.

> I think diabetes for me – well it did take a lot of the pleasure away, took a lot of the: 'it's my body' – 'it's my pregnancy' [away from me].

In some instances this dissatisfaction led to (and was probably influenced by) problematic relationships with health care professionals. This was particularly relevant when women felt themselves to be under close surveillance and some women reported feeling infantilized, for example:

> Sometimes it's the person that you're seeing as well, if you don't have a good rapport … I'd just felt sometimes like I was a naughty schoolgirl, and I used to dread putting some of the [blood-glucose] readings in my diary.

> … the doctor I encountered was awful – he was hideous – a most vile man and I walked out crying and I just thought, well how dare he tell me what I will and won't do! … You won't eat this, you won't eat that, you know what I mean? Particularly in the early stages of pregnancy when you're throwing up and you have a dietician saying, 'you can't eat this' and this is the only thing you can keep down.

> … sometimes I was spoken to like I was a piece of crap on the floor … and I felt like … well you are telling me things here that I know and that are not the situation.

Lawson and Rajaram (1994) noted that women with diabetes in pregnancy struggled with the various possible definitions of their pregnancy as 'normal', 'abnormal' or 'illness'. Persson, Winkvist and Mogren (2010) describe women with gestational diabetes as being 'stunned', and highlight the loss of a sense of normality, both in terms of the loss of a 'normal' pregnancy, as well as the loss of normal lifestyle. Most apparent in our discussion groups was recognition that the management of diabetes spoiled the notion of a happy, normal pregnancy free of problems and complications, as the following two women indicate:

> It [the diabetes] just dominates the pregnancy all the way through, takes all the joy out of it.

> Immediately you become high risk – it's in your notes. You'll probably be… induced early and it just changes everything so quickly.

All the women we spoke to, regardless of their type of diabetes, reported feeling that the health care professionals' over-riding concern was with their diabetes, in particular blood glucose levels and insulin treatment, at the expense of a more positive experience of pregnancy and childbirth. A Swedish study of diabetes in pregnancy noted similarly that: 'The healthy parts of the pregnancy had been forced into the background and there was too much focus on diabetes … [this] easily can be overlooked and especially when a disease is present' (Anderberg, Berntorp and Crang-Svalenius 2009: 166-8).

Some of the women in the discussion groups had attended diabetes ante-natal clinics that were jointly run between the diabetologist and the obstetrician, and these were perceived positively because of improved communication between health care professionals.

Many of the women reported only seeing health care professionals in hospitals and did not have access to a community midwife during pregnancy. Not only did this reinforce the medicalized nature of their pregnancy, it also engendered feelings of isolation as they spent their time in large busy hospital clinics, rather than at smaller, local settings in the community where women with low risk pregnancies are seen. This segregation added to feelings of being 'different' from other pregnant women who were experiencing a 'normal' pregnancy; a finding also noted by Thomas (2003) in her study of pregnancy and chronic illness.

To summarize, whilst experiences of diabetes in pregnancy are not all the same, the women who participated in our discussion groups highlighted a tension between the medical management of diabetes and the experience of pregnancy, the former of these being prioritized by health professionals in the delivery of care. Women seem to need a greater emphasis on the experience of being pregnant, seeking to emphasise the 'normal' and 'natural' aspects of the experience rather than those associated with the increased surveillance and monitoring of a medical condition. It is this very juxtaposition of anticipated normalcy against the medicalization of the pregnancy which presents a loss of expectations for women during pregnancy.

Care during Labour and Delivery

In contrast to experiences of care in pregnancy, where the women felt that there was too much emphasis on managing diabetes at the expense of other dimensions of their pregnancies, in labour, some of the women felt that further support from specialist diabetes care staff would have been helpful. For example, two participants commented on this:

> My insulin drip came out and no one seemed sure whether they should put I back in or not.

> When you're in labour … it would have been nice to have a diabetes nurse or doctor to reassure you that everything's alright … although I had the drip in I don't remember anyone talking to me about my diabetes.

Similar findings were noted by Anderberg, Berntorp and Crang-Svalenius who argue that: 'This focus on diabetes was relevant for all areas of care except for delivery department, where the situation was reversed. The women felt that focus there was predominantly on the normal and experienced that responsibility for the control's necessary for their diabetes rested heavily on them.' (2009: 166). Whilst the joint diabetes/obstetric service during pregnancy was seen as a positive aspect of service development, the same could not be said in relation to women's experiences of labour Indeed, one of the women in our discussion groups felt that she needed to remind staff that she had diabetes:

> Although they were aware of it I had to keep reminding them. 'Oh is it OK to have these?' I had nothing to eat.

In their study of experiences of support during pregnancy and childbirth of women with Type 1 diabetes, Berg and Sparud-Lundin (2009) also found that women felt abandoned during childbirth when it came to managing glycaemic control. Indeed, little information had been given to the women to prepare them for the possible consequences of diabetes for childbirth, as one woman commented:

> I don't think I even thought that it would make any difference to my labour. Not at all, I don't remember them saying they would test me during the labour or anything. Because I hadn't been through it before, I didn't know what to expect. But I know for next time, I'm guaranteed to get diabetes again so I'm booking in for a c-section!

Here, a gap between information received from diabetologists and information from midwives and obstetricians – as well as a lack of communication within the health care team – was in evidence, highlighting the differences between different teams and professions, as well as between generalists and specialists. A lack of joined up care has also been identified by another team of researchers in Sweden (Berg and Sparud-Lundin 2009) who suggest that women are often the ones that communicate between health professionals because information is not effectively shared between members of health care teams.

Childbirth is often described as a joyful, even empowering experience, albeit a painful one. However, even the pain of childbirth has been described in positive terms in anticipation of a happy event: a live and healthy baby. The data presented here, and other literature, suggest that childbirth experiences can be marred by the way in which women are expected to take responsibility for managing their diabetes during labour and delivery even if they are not really equipped to do so.

During pregnancy, diabetes is at the fore of medical care but during childbirth the reverse is true.

Care after Childbirth

Data from the discussion groups suggest that in the immediate post-natal period, women are expected to take responsibility for their diabetes even when they do not necessarily have the knowledge or experience to do so. In contrast to the pride of place diabetes has during pregnancy, after birth (as during labour), diabetes is neglected, as one participant comments here:

> On the post-natal ward when my blood sugar was so high, nobody there knew why it was and what to do about it … you've got a new baby who needs attention but your blood sugars are through the roof…

As reported by Sparud-Lundin and Berg (2011) in their Swedish study, health professionals may reinforce women's feelings of vulnerability during early motherhood since they (like women themselves) may have insufficient knowledge about managing diabetes, or may appear unconcerned or ignorant.

A number of the women in our discussion groups also reported some distress after being separated from their baby immediately after the birth, or very shortly after, when they were sent to neonatal care for further monitoring. Sparud-Lundin and Berg (2011) suggest that women's vulnerability following childbirth can be reinforced in the early post-partum period when women and babies are separated. Two of the participants talked about being separated from their baby:

> … we did have her for about an hour … that was hard there were three women with their babies crying all night (in the ward room she shared) then there's me. I felt like I didn't have a baby.

> Then someone took him under the arms and he left. I thought where has he gone? … they got someone from special care they said the baby didn't register on the scale so we have to take him away so we had a quick cuddle and he was gone. He was gone … So that was a weird experience.

Another participant compares her recent experience of being able to stay with her baby to a former experience where her baby was taken into neonatal care:

> Yes when I had my first about two hours after he was born they tested his sugars and it had dropped so they whisked him off to the special care unit where he was for two to three days. But they do it differently now – just come and test her – I think it is every couple of hours and she can stay with me and that is so much [better]. When you think you have gone through the pregnancy, people testing

> your blood all the time, it was lovely being able to keep the baby with me rather than being taken away and that is a new thing as I say and that was much better.

The CEMACH report, *Diabetes in Pregnancy: Caring for baby after birth* (2007) revealed that in more than 50 per cent of women with Type 1 and Type 2 diabetes, babies are automatically moved to neonatal care when there is no specific medical indication for admission. The report goes on to suggest that hospitals should be encouraging early interaction between mothers and babies unless there are contraindications and not simply separating women from infants because it is 'hospital policy'. Thus, women with diabetes are far more likely to experience the immediate removal of their infant into neonatal care than are women without diabetes, and the subsequent losses that arise from this in relation to early interaction.

The same report (CEMACH 2007) also highlights the impact of diabetes on breastfeeding, noting that a quarter of babies were not fed early enough and that two thirds of babies were given infant formula as a first feed. The report is conclusive in arguing that there is no reason for women with diabetes not to breastfeed, should this be their choice. Some of the women in our discussion groups felt undermined when trying to breastfeed in hospital:

> … I explained that I was stressed and they made me sit there and breast feed her in front of them to make sure I was doing it right. Now when I think back I don't know why I didn't say, 'Oh just get stuffed', but your hormones are everywhere.

> They came in didn't say anything just took her blood sugars, they just came with this bottle said 'is this OK?'. I said no because I'm breastfeeding her, they said they had to because her blood sugars were low, I was quite upset about this … I wanted to breastfeed her but because her blood sugars were low they were giving her formula and they said that I had to give her formula to get her blood sugars up. And then it took four, five weeks to get her feeding off me and it was just such a trauma …

Other studies have highlighted how the initiation of breastfeeding is an important part of the transition to motherhood. However, the data from this and other studies suggest that little support is available in the immediate post-natal period to support breastfeeding particularly in the context of managing blood-glucose levels (Rasmussen et al. 2007, Sparud-Lundin and Berg 2011). So, whilst not all women will choose to breastfeed, and women without diabetes may also struggle to receive the support they need to initiate and maintain breastfeeding, women with diabetes have an additional burden since they must negotiate this within the context of their experience of diabetes.

Diabetes can also have a significant impact on women's future plans regarding pre-conception care, pregnancy management, expectations around labour, delivery and the post-natal period. Planning for future fertility and family size was also an issue. In the quote below one of the participants with pre-existing diabetes describes her feelings:

> I got pregnant after having 12 miscarriages. I think the preconception frightened me a little bit, and we did question, are we going to bother doing this? 'Cause I think it was the horror stories, the risk of stillborns and all this, you just start thinking, 'can I really put myself through all this'?

In the next two quotes, women with GDM talk about their anxieties in relation to possible future pregnancies:

> I know if I had known … well what seriously put me off having another baby would be the insulin. The first time wasn't too bad – I was about 30 weeks pregnant so that wasn't too bad and it was OK with the diet – but this time they seemed to jump in so quick with the insulin and I kept says' no, no I'm not going on insulin until I have really got to …

> It didn't affect me with Hannah as it [GDM] was only picked up in the last 8 weeks, but with this one it was from week 8 – it kind of takes over your whole life so yes I'd think carefully about a third one.

In the final quote below, one participant describes the impact of diabetes on other people and in this instance, on her husband:

> …with the second one, I was more concerned because I knew what had happened during the first. And my husband saying, never again, I never want us to go through that again, but we did and he was petrified. I know, at the beginning of the pregnancy, he used to phone five or six times a day because, I mean, he used to come home and find me unconscious with the second time pregnancy, I thought he was going to leave me he was so absolutely petrified at what he was going to come home and find.

So, in the immediate post-natal period the data from the discussion groups presented here suggest that – as experienced during childbirth – women themselves are often expected to take responsibility for managing their diabetes, diverting attention from the transition to motherhood, recovery from labour and delivery and early interaction with their baby. Women with diabetes are also more likely to have their baby taken into neonatal care, and may experience more difficulties – for a variety of reasons – in establishing breastfeeding. All of these events can be experienced as a form of loss. In addition to this, diabetes can influence women's decisions regarding their future fertility, and can have an effect on other family members.

Final Thoughts on the Pregnancy Paradox

There is a fairly limited social sciences literature on diabetes in pregnancy, although its application can shed light on the impact of this condition on experiences of pregnancy, birth and early motherhood (Stenhouse and Letherby 2011). Our data, and other literature, suggest that a chronic illness such as diabetes can impact significantly on women's experiences of pregnancy, leaving some women feeling infantilized, under surveillance and overly medicalized. It would seem that women are deprived of the many simple pleasures of pregnancy because as one of the participants clearly states, the experience is 'more about the diabetes than the pregnancy.' Whilst not all experiences are negative by any means, and there are many examples of good care, there is an overall loss of the sense of normality. In being diagnosed with diabetes or defined as high risk there is also the loss of a normal lifestyle, with restrictions on diet, requirements to monitor blood-glucose levels and the need to attend regular medical appointments in what might be a large, unfamiliar setting. In labour and in the immediate post-natal period, an expectation that women will manage their diabetes, even though they may not be equipped to do so, also contributes to the loss of a sense of normality. For some women, this experience is compounded further when their baby is removed to neonatal care or they experience difficulties in establishing breastfeeding because of their diabetes. The impact of diabetes on future reproductive decision-making is also important as negative experiences, the fear of administering insulin or the fear of infant mortality or morbidity can have consequences for women and their families. For some women this implies a loss of the idealized notion of trouble-free pregnancy, whereas other women may feel the need to curtail desired future pregnancies.

Women with diabetes in pregnancy are not a homogenous group. Some women will have had diabetes from a very young age, whereas others will develop diabetes in their early adult years before pregnancy. This form of diabetes is often associated with being obese or overweight, but it is also more common in women who are from minority ethnic groups, as well as those who live in deprivation. Other women will develop diabetes for the first time during pregnancy and this is sometimes detected early on in a pregnancy but, for other women, it sometimes develops, or is detected just shortly before delivery. These differences influence women's experiences and the extent to which diabetes in pregnancy is experienced as a form of reproductive loss. Regardless of this heterogeneity, pregnancy, childbirth and early motherhood are experienced paradoxically against a backdrop of anticipated normalcy, where all women will be, and want to be mothers, where all pregnancies are wanted and successful, and where experiences of the pregnancy process are expected to be happy and fulfilling (Earle and Letherby 2003).

References

Anderberg, E., Berntorp, K. and Crang-Svalenius, E. 2009. Diabetes and pregnancy: women's opinions about the care provided during the childbearing year. *Scandinavian Journal of Caring Sciences*, 23, 161-170.

Barahona, M.J., Sucunza, N., Garcia-Patterson, A., Hernandez, M., Adelantado, J.M., Ginovart, G., De Leiva, A. and Corcoy, R. 2005. Period of gestational diabetes mellitus diagnosis and maternal and fetal morbidity. *Acta Obstetrica et Gynecologica Scandinavica*, 84(7), 622-627.

Berg, M. and Sparud-Lundin, C. 2009. Experiences of professional support during pregnancy and childbirth – a qualitative study of women with type I diabetes. *BMC Pregnancy and Childbirth*, 9(27), Available at: http://www.biomedcentral.com/1471-2393/9/27 [accessed: 11 July 2011].

Bury, M. 1982. Chronic illness as biographical disruption. *Sociology of Health & Illness*, 4, 167-182.

Casson, I.F. 2006. Pregnancy in women with diabetes – after the CEMACH report, what now? *Diabetic Medicine*, 23, 481-484.

CEMACH. 2007. *Confidential Enquiry into Maternal and Child Health. Diabetes in Pregnancy: Are we Providing the Best Care?* London: CEMACH.

CEMACH. 2007. *Diabetes in Pregnancy: Caring for baby after birth.* London: CEMACH.

CEMACH. 2010. *Confidential Enquiry into Maternal and Child Health (CEMACH). Perinatal Mortality 2008.* London: CEMACH.

Cotterill, P. 1994. *Friendly relations? Mothers and their daughters-in-law.* London: Taylor & Francis.

Coulthard. T., Hawthorne, G., on behalf of the Northern Diabetes Pregnancy Service. 2008. Type 2 diabetes in pregnancy; more to come? *Practical Diabetes International*, 25(9), 359-361.

Earle, S. and Letherby, G. (eds) 2003. *Gender, Identity and Reproduction: Social Perspectives*. London: Palgrave.

Earle, S., Foley, P., Komaromy, C. and Lloyd, C. 2008. Conceptualising reproductive loss: A social sciences perspective. *Human Fertility*, 11(4), 259-262.

Evans, M. and O'Brien, B. 2005. Gestational diabetes: The meaning of an at-risk pregnancy. *Qualitative Health Research*, 15(66), 66-81.

Exley, C. and Letherby, G. 2001. Managing a disrupted lifecourse: Issues of identity and emotion work. *Health*, 5, 112-132.

Goffman, E. 1968. *Asylums: Essays on the Social Situation of Mental Patients and Other Inmates.* New York: Anchor Books.

Hockey, J. and James, A. 1993. *Growing Up and Growing Old: Ageing and Dependency in the Lifecourse*. London: Sage.

Jobling, R. 1977. Learning to live with it: an account of a career of chronic dermatological illness and patienthood, in *Medical Encounters: The experience of illness and treatment*, edited by A. Davis and G. Horobin. London: Croom Helm, 72-86.

Lawson, E.J. and Rajaram, S. 1994. A transformed pregnancy: the psychosocial consequences of gestational diabetes. *Sociology of Health & Illness*, 16(4), 536-62.

Layne, L.L. 2003. Unhappy endings: A feminist reappraisal of the women's health movement from the vantage of pregnancy loss. *Social Science & Medicine*, 56, 1881-1891.

Lloyd, C.E., Underwood, L., Winkley, K., Nouwen, A., Hermanns, N. and Pouwer, F. 2010. The epidemiology of diabetes and depression in *Depression and Diabetes*, edited by W. Katon, M. Maj and N. Sartorius. Oxford: Wiley/Blackwell.

National Institute of Health and Clinical Excellence. (NICE). 2008. *Diabetes in Pregnancy: management of diabetes and its complications from pre-conception to the post-natal period.* Clinical guideline 63, London: NICE. Available at: http://www.nice.org.uk/nicemedia/live/11946/41320/41320.pdf [accessed 11 July 2011].

Persson, M., Hörnsten, A., Winkvist, A. and Mogren, I. 2011. 'Mission impossible?' Midwives' experiences counseling pregnant women with gestational diabetes mellitus. *Patient Education and Counseling*, 84, 78-83.

Persson, M., Winkvist, A. and Mogren, I. 2009. 'From stun to gradual balance' – women's experiences of living with gestational diabetes mellitus. *Scandinavian Journal of Caring Sciences*, 24, 454-462.

Rasmussen, B., O'Connell, B., Dunning, P. and Cox, H. 2007. Young women with Type 1 diabetes; management of turning points and transitions. *Qualitative Health Research*, 17, 300-310.

Sparud-Lundin, C. and Merg, M. 2011. Extraordinary exposed in early motherhood – a qualitative study exploring experiences of mothers with Type 1 diabetes, *BMC Women's Health*, 11(10). Available at: http://www.biomedcentral.com/1472-6874/11/10 [accessed 7 July 2011].

Stenhouse, E. and Letherby, G. 2011. Mother/daughter relationships during pregnancy and the transition to motherhood of women with pre-existing diabetes: raising some issues. *Midwifery*, 27, 120-124.

Thomas, H. 2003. Pregnancy, illness and the concept of career. *Sociology of Health & Illness*, 25(5), 383-407.

Watts, S., O'Hara, L. and Trigg, R. 2010. Living with Type 1 diabetes: A by-person qualitative exploration. *Psychology & Health*, 25(4), 491-506.

Chapter 6

'Silent' Miscarriage and Deafening Heteronormativity: A British Experiential and Critical Feminist Account

Elizabeth Peel and Ruth Cain

In this chapter we provide a critical feminist analysis of sonographically-diagnosed miscarriage, otherwise known as 'silent', 'missed' or delayed miscarriage, using our experiential accounts as a catalyst to explore both academic and lay literatures surrounding pregnancy loss. We delineate the similarities and differences in our own experiences (one of us part of a lesbian married couple; the other part of a heterosexual married couple) before focusing on relational context as a prime site of difference. Through an examination of scholarly and 'self-help' writing on miscarriage we argue that pervasive heteronormativity doubly marginalises the experiences of lesbians – and women otherwise located outside the realm of heterosexual relationships. In conclusion, we suggest a more thorough engagement with 'non-normative' experiences of pregnancy loss will substantially enhance our understandings of miscarriage. Placing marginalised experience and non-normative groups of women more firmly within pregnancy loss scholarship promises to significantly augment critical, feminist and social scientific theorising. This more expansive consideration of the diversity of women's lives and experiences is also likely to help pregnancy loss become included in reproductive health agendas.

Pregnancy loss is an example of the cultural silence around reproductive 'malfunction': statistically common, it remains shrouded in secrecy (Renner et al. 2000). Early loss (before 20 weeks gestation) occurs in between 15 to 31 per cent of confirmed pregnancies (Cosgrove 2004). Yet the normative western narrative of pregnancy is continually reproduced: a missed period, a positive home pregnancy test, and a medically managed pregnancy prominently featuring visits to view the developing 'baby' via ultrasound (Davis-Floyd and Dumit 1998). Pregnancy loss at any stage of gestation 'does not conform to the norm' of joyful maternity, and represents 'an incomplete rite of passage' for women in the normative route to motherhood (Layne 2003: 27, 39). It also contradicts medical norms of correct reproductive embodiment, since it exposes and disrupts the myth of linear 'biomedical progress' implicit in western 'technobirthing' discourses, which make pregnancy and child-rearing the object of rationalizing medical interventions and management (Layne 2003: 176).

Silent miscarriage occurs when the foetus dies in utero and is discovered by ultrasound scan before the foetus is expelled. In other words, as far as women are concerned, until the loss is diagnosed by sonogram the pregnancy appears to be progressing. This was the type of loss experienced by both authors. Although the term missed miscarriage is more commonly used to describe this experience in, for instance, widely accessed internet resources such as babycentre.co.uk (Hammonds 2009), we prefer silent miscarriage as this term conveys the cultural silence around miscarriage as well as the lack of clear physiological symptoms of loss and the comparative rarity of this type of miscarriage. Of course, this particular form of pregnancy loss is dependent upon the availability, frequency, and point of use of sonograms within any given pregnancy trajectory. We have not been able to locate published statistics on the frequency of silent miscarriage – a fact that partly reflects the lack of attention paid to the subjective and bodily experience of pregnancy loss, which clearly alters when the miscarriage is discovered in this way. It also reflects national differences in the prevalence and use of ultrasound. In Britain the first routine ultrasound is offered to National Health Service (NHS) patients at around 12 weeks into pregnancy unless there have been previous antenatal problems, in which case an aptly named 'viability scan' is offered at around eight weeks. Women with the resources to do so also have the choice of paying for an earlier private scan. In the USA, the frequency of silent miscarriage will be higher as a routine first scan is at 8 weeks (Swain and Layne 2005). Indeed in cultures where ultrasound technologies aren't available this specific form of pregnancy loss, shaped as it is by medical technologies, doesn't exist. But as Layne (1992) highlights there is always dis-synchronicity in pregnancy loss – a lag between demise and expulsion from the body. In Peel's (2010) online survey of British, American, Canadian and Australian lesbian and bisexual women's experience of pregnancy loss 36 per cent of participants found out about their loss through ultrasound, but as this was a convenience sample no conclusions about prevalence can be drawn. We can speculate, however, that the fairly high number of losses revealed in this way partly reflects the relatively high usage of assisted reproduction technologies (ARTs) including ultrasound in this sample (Peel 2010).

Moreover, the narrative of normal pregnancy begins with 'natural' conception within a heterosexual relationship, usually marriage. Lesbian motherhood is less common than heterosexual motherhood, and lesbian routes to conception are by definition non-(hetero) normative. Furthermore, since most lesbians use ARTs (insemination with known or anonymous donor sperm) or adopt children, their family-forming practices are also likely to be considered non-normative. Even in cases where no medical assistance is used for conception, lesbian pregnancies are prone to classification as 'artificial' (Ferrara, Ballet and Grudzinkas 2000, Mamo 2007).

Statistics on the number of lesbian mothers are vague. About one third of British lesbians are mothers (Golombok et al. 2003). And even less is known about the incidence of pregnancy loss among lesbian women. A study of intrauterine insemination with frozen donor sperm (122 single heterosexual women and 35 lesbian couples attending a fertility clinic in London) found that in 63 pregnancies the miscarriage rate was 15 per cent for lesbian couples and 35 per cent for single heterosexual women (Ferrara, Balet and Grudzinkas 2000). The authors suggest that the difference in miscarriage rates between the two groups may be due to the heterosexual single women in their study being older than the lesbians; having failed to conceive for some time prior to clinic referral. Examining sonographically-diagnosed early pregnancy loss is important for a number of reasons. First, research suggests women's feelings about miscarriage are not influenced by gestational age at loss (Swanson et al. 2007, Cosgrove 2004), and so first trimester miscarriage can be just as distressing as later pregnancy loss or stillbirth. Second, there are particular nuances of silent miscarriage that increase the prospective parents' sense of 'fetal personhood' (Layne 2003: 101, Petchesky 1987), since the death of the foetus is experienced later than it physiologically occurred; an unintended consequence of a new reproductive technology. While sonography has been well studied by interdisciplinary feminist scholars of the new reproductive technologies (for example see Harpel 2008), this unintended consequence has been almost entirely neglected. The medical benefits of routine sonography in pregnancy and the great pleasure that many women and their families take in 'seeing the baby' and sharing the baby with others that this affords outweigh any consideration for the many women who will learn they have lost their pregnancy this way. As one British lesbian in Peel's (2010: 725) study vividly expresses: 'I get very angry that people see this [ultrasound] as an opportunity to put the first photo in the album not as a serious medical procedure with potentially disastrous news'.

Furthermore, as Peel (2010: 725) reports 'numbness, shock, distress and devastation were the overriding emotions conveyed by those respondents who had their loss revealed to them in this way'. As one of her survey respondents – a self-labelled butch dyke from the USA – elucidated:

> We were very excited going for an ultrasound at our obstetrician's office – so far the pregnancy seemed to be going well – I was having symptoms but none of them were too extreme. My wife Emma was a medical student so she was a little more cautious than me knowing that many things can go wrong this early in a pregnancy – I really expected any kind of pregnancy loss to be symptomatic and since I hadn't had any cramping or bleeding at all I didn't expect there to be any problems … Emma started crying and I just felt really numb. (Peel 2010: 725)

Another respondent, a British bisexual woman, was 'absolutely devastated' and found it 'enormously, terribly distressing' (725) to have first one and then subsequently a second pregnancy loss revealed through sonogram.

With reference to social science and 'self-help' literature, including our own experiences, this chapter explores the non-normative experience and consequences of silent miscarriage. While not an autoethnographic analysis per se (c.f., Sheach Leith 2009, Ellis 2004), our argument is embedded in experiential perspectives. We focus particularly on how lesbians' experiences of pregnancy loss are marginalised within an overarching context of heteronormative, 'natural' pregnancy (Peel 2010). Attention to pregnancy loss in such marginal contexts could help to refocus medical and psychological practice on the varying needs of each woman in this traumatic situation. Also, it could broaden feminist concepts of the embodied 'standpoint' of the reproducing woman, whether she is a socially, legally and clinically recognized 'mother', 'mother-without-child', 'non-mother', or 'would-have-been mother' (Hansen 1997).

Experiential Accounts of Silent Miscarriage

Both Liz and Ruth had the shared experience of shock and dissociation in finding out, in the coldly technical setting of an ultrasound room during their first sonogram, that, to quote the health professionals involved, their pregnancies were not 'viable'. Liz's pregnancy loss occurred within the context of a planned lesbian parent family. Ruth was heterosexually married and her pregnancy was unplanned. Below we recount our experiences of pregnancy and loss.

Liz's Story, 2008

> We started the conception process in the autumn of 2007. Five months later Rosie (my wife) and I were becoming disillusioned and less believing that a minute amount of liquid in a syringe could enable us to have a baby. I did everything as the books suggested – even slowly rotating myself so the sperm would coat my entire cervix. Each month we waited, hoped, tested, waited a while longer, tested again and then my period arrived and we'd go through the process of checking, negotiating, coordinating and collecting sperm from our friend again. After I'd convinced myself getting pregnant wasn't going to work for me I conceived in March 2008.
>
> Rosie and I were thrilled I was pregnant and told family and friends immediately. We bought a new family home with room for a nursery, and the baby clothes and shoes that couldn't be resisted; evaluated different cots and buggies and agreed on a name. The fact that I wasn't sick didn't trouble me. I could compare notes with my also pregnant (and very sick) sister and feel secretly self-congratulatory – all the organic vegetables, herbal teas and vitamins were elevating me above the realms of morning sickness. We were very excited about the routine 12 week scan – it meant being able to tell people at work – and we needn't be concerned with the possibility of miscarriage any more, the books said. I'd noticed some dark blood the week before and anxiously called the midwife (no answer) so I phoned the hospital where we were due to have the scan and spoke to a receptionist who said someone would call me back. But they never did. Surely they would have returned my call if there was anything to worry about? And in

any case, I'd heard that women can 'spot' throughout their pregnancy and the blood I'd seen wasn't fresh so it couldn't be problematic.

We attended the scan appointment at the maternity department of the local hospital. As instructed, I made sure I had a full bladder for the ultrasound and we organized the five pound coins we needed in order to get a ticket which would be exchanged for the scan picture of our baby. There was this cataclysmic disjuncture between our excited expectation and the unfolding experience. The sonographer looked concerned and from the looming chasm of disbelief I was slipping into came the words: *'there doesn't appear to be a heartbeat'; 'there's a foetal pole and sac'; 'this is the worst part of my job' and 'failed pregnancy'.* But there must have been some uncertainty because another sonographer was brought in and I was vaginally probed.

Ruth's Story, 2002

My husband and I looked forward to the 12 week scan, when we would see 'our baby'. We told everyone well before the scan date; congratulations were ours in abundance. The fact that I felt no sickness confirmed my belief that I could breeze through pregnancy. After all, I had become pregnant so easily.

I had begun to bleed slightly the day before; no cramps. Bleeding, I read on the internet, was a sign of miscarriage in 50 per cent of cases. Something could well be wrong; but I felt the bleeding was too light to mean anything.

At the scan, my husband focused on the screen before us. The scan technician grinned at his eager face. A poster in the waiting room showed a cartoon foetus complete with wiggly umbilical cord, shouting to *'mum': 'if you want a photo of me, tell the technician before you leave!'*. The technician stopped smiling and turned the screen away. I felt a dull recognition of defeat settle upon me: *'I'm sorry, I can't see a heartbeat.'* It had seemed to slump to the bottom of the womb. It had a shrimplike shape, with something like arms seeming to emerge from its tiny torso.

The trajectory of the 'baby's' existence did not end at its predicted birth date. On the day the pregnancy calendars gave for its birth, I found I was pregnant with my now eight year old son. The anxiety attached to the miscarried foetus fastened itself firmly upon its successor.

There are similarities in both stories: the medicalized experience, treatment by the NHS, emotional reactions and subsequent grief, and joy at our subsequent children. There are also axes of difference. Liz experienced her loss in 2008 and Ruth in 2002. Liz was treated in a regional town, Ruth in London. Another difference, which we now go onto explore more broadly, is how our relational contexts shaped these experiences. In other words, we offer a critical evaluation of how being in same-sex versus different-sex relationships affects the experience of pregnancy loss. We begin by outlining the invisibility of lesbians in the pregnancy (and pregnancy loss) literature before discussing the management of miscarriage.

Lesbians and Pregnancy Loss: Doubly Invisible

Lesbians and bisexual women are all but invisible in the generic literatures on pregnancy and pregnancy loss. The 'heterosexist monopoly of reproduction' (Wojnar and Swanson 2006: 5) is invidiously pervasive (Mamo 2007). Popular pregnancy and childbirth books (and the literature presented to women by general practitioners (GPs) and midwives after confirmation of pregnancy) in the UK are similarly heteronormative. (See for example 'Emma's Diary', the pregnancy guidance booklet written in fictional diary form and distributed by GPs to pregnant women who have contact with antenatal services [Royal College of General Practitioners 1997].) British anthropologist Sheila Kitzinger devotes four of her 448 pages in *The New Pregnancy and Childbirth* to miscarriage, to a chapter entitled (insensitively in this context) 'You and your newborn'. Lesbians do not receive a mention, even in passing. The very popular 421-page British book *Rough Guide to Pregnancy and Birth* (Cooke 2001) dedicates just over two pages to miscarriage in the chapter focused on 'Week 6'. Again, there is no mention of lesbians in the book. A best-selling American manual, *What to Expect When You're Expecting* (Eisenberg, Murkow and Hathaway 1991) makes no mention of same sex parenting and mentions miscarriage very briefly. The absence of lesbian parents in this very normative popular literature parallels that of lone parents (female or male) and non-normative conception methods.

In the dedicated lesbian pregnancy self-help literature, discussion of pregnancy loss is similarly lacking. However, in a book entitled *The Essential Guide to Lesbian Conception, Pregnancy, and Birth* written by American midwives (Toevs and Brill 2002) just six of 487 pages discuss miscarriage.

Toevs and Brill (2002: 395) acknowledge that 'because of the lack of openness surrounding its normalcy, miscarriage has become unnecessarily medicalized' and recognize that 'pregnancy loss is a big marker in women's lives'. They note two ways that miscarriage poses special challenges for lesbians' writing: 'While in the crisis, you may also need to decide how to represent your family structure, and you may have to filter through the possible homophobia or judgments about single mothers, which, more than likely, will only add to your stress' (396). They also mention how the difficulty of becoming pregnant for lesbians affects grief. Whereas, heterosexually married women bridle when told, 'oh you can always have another one'. Such a suggestion is more thoughtless to women (regardless of their sexuality) who have gone through the process of sperm acquisition and artificial insemination: 'Grieving takes on an additional dimension when you realize you're basically starting all over when you inseminate again' (398). Lisa Saffron (2001), the British lesbian mother, writer and activist provides one page on miscarriage in her 331 page book *It's a Family Affair: The Complete Lesbian Parenting Book*, in a chapter entitled 'when it doesn't go as planned'. She also provides the story of a would-be lesbian mother entitled 'A lost dream – Casey's story' (109-113). Casey describes her multiple miscarriages including one that she learned of during her scan: 'Before the scan with the first miscarriage she [her partner Lesley] had been concerned, while I had not seriously considered that pregnancy loss could be a possibility' (112). This is the only mention of a lesbian's miscarriages discovered by a scan we have been able to find in the 'self-help' literature.

Feminist scholarship is little better on the subject of pregnancy loss in non-heteronormative contexts. For example, in Layne's (2003) feminist anthropology of pregnancy loss in America, she never addresses lesbians. Indeed, Celia Kitzinger's (1996) idiom of 'the token lesbian chapter' coined in the context of feminist psychology over fifteen years ago seems utopian when applied to the pregnancy loss literature. The 'tokenism' of feminism in relation to lesbian parenting disturbingly mirrors the exclusionary tendencies of mainstream pregnancy literature which occludes 'abnormal' narratives of pregnancy or parenthood. As Lisa Cosgrove (2004: 113) highlights in her feminist critique of the academic pregnancy loss literature:

> Despite awareness that technological advances have allowed many women to get pregnant who previously would not have been able to, the voices of single or lesbian mothers and non-traditional couples are nowhere to be found in the research literature. By failing to consider the ways in which implicit assumptions about compulsory heterosexuality determine the focus of their work, researchers have actively silenced the experiences of many women and their partners … [this] must be addressed so that 'women's responses' to pregnancy loss are not conflated with 'married heterosexual women's responses to pregnancy loss.

Empirical research about lesbians' experiences of pregnancy loss is scant. Only two studies to date have focused on non-heterosexual women's experiences (Peel 2010, Wojnar 2007). Wojnar (2007) conducted a phenomenological study based on 10 interviews with white US lesbian couples. She found that the participants who were growing the baby (which she describes as birth mothers) typically bonded with the unborn child very early in pregnancy and that they grieved their loss openly, whilst the non-pregnant participants, social mothers, kept their sadness more private, feeling that they needed to be strong for their partners, much as men in heterosexual couples are reported to do (Puddifoot and Johnson 1997). Wojnar (2007: 483) concluded that: 'in contrast with heterosexuals whose unintended pregnancy rates linger at about 50 per cent, lesbian pregnancies are generally planned and wanted … regardless of how long it took couples to conceive, the 'typical' stressful process of becoming pregnant for lesbians was similar to the 'atypical' experience of the subset of heterosexual women who experience infertility'. Similarly, Peel's more recent research based on online survey responses from 60 non-heterosexual women from the UK, USA, Canada and Australia found that the experience of loss was amplified due to participants' relational situations, and the financial and emotional investment respondents had made in order to achieve conception (Peel 2010).

Miscarriage (Mis)Management

Regardless of our sexual orientations, we both received horrible 'care'. Our emotional losses and physical pain were minimised and ignored.

> Liz: Three weeks after the scan that revealed the 'failed pregnancy' I was given The Miscarriage Association's 'We're sorry that you have had a miscarriage' leaflet by a hospital midwife. I said they really should provide information earlier as I didn't have a clue what to expect, and was told it would be like a 'heavy period'. She replied platitudinally 'we'll take that on board'. During the worst of the bleeding and clots I experienced horrific pain. That was my experience of 'expectantly managed' miscarriage (see also Cote-Arsenault, Scare and Layne, 2006; Layne, 2006, 2007, Maclean and Layne 2006).

> Ruth: We sat in Accident and Emergency (A&E or Emergency Room) for three hours. I then remember the blank face of the doctor who examined me in a windowless room; she stood back and looked at the wall as I burst into tears of shock. She concluded her examination with the news that to avoid infection, I must return for an operation: 'the products of conception must be removed'. The phrase was the ugliest I had ever heard.

The female body, particularly in 'abnormal' reproductive contexts, is a disciplinary site. Medicalisation, pathologising and legal control of 'unruly' bodies all play their parts in the production and maintenance of femininity (Ussher 1991, Foucault 1990). The 'power' exercised here is not unipolar and totalitarian, but patchy and variable (Foucault 1980). Our stories provide anecdotal examples of such variability, over a relatively brief time period (2002-2008) and in different areas of the UK. Ruth was given no option but to undergo an Evacuation of Retained Products of Conception (ERPC) procedure involving a general anaesthetic in 2002. In 2008 Liz was told to 'wait and see' (otherwise referred to as 'expectant management', see also Layne, 2006). Medical management of miscarriage changed during the last decade of the twentieth century and the six-year gap between our experiences reflects this: there is now a tendency to allow 'expectant management' rather than opting automatically for a surgical solution (Nanda et al. 2006, Griebel et al. 2005). 'Expectant management' allows the body to miscarry in its own time, although it should be noted that this will not always happen and that there are risks attached to both forms of management (Jauniaux, Johns and Burton 2005, Sotiriadis et al. 2005, Wieringa-de Waard et al. 2003). ERPC is associated with a higher risk of infection (Nanda et al. 2006) and while the anxiety associated with surgery is avoided in 'expectant management', the latter involves much pain, bleeding and knowingly carrying a dead foetus for days or weeks.

Perhaps more importantly, the risks and benefits of each kind of management appear to be inadequately represented to women. The research literature emphasizes 'the woman's preference' (for example, Nanda et al. 2006, Smith et al. 2006), but in both cases we were given no options at all, and scant information from which to make any independent choice or judgment (see further Smith et al. 2006).

An important aspect of the silencing of miscarriage experience is that of emotional suppression, the unacceptability of grief for the loss. Medical care for women in Britain is routinely criticised for being perfunctory, insensitive, and unsupportive, and aftercare barely exists (Nikcevic 2003). Society (including both heterosexuals and lesbians) fails to recognise grief, particularly for losses in early pregnancy (women are routinely told to 'just try again' for a baby); and in Britain there is also too little professional support, women and their partners tend to suffer alone. Professional awareness of, and training in, the psychological issues surrounding early pregnancy loss and its aftermath appears to be minimal despite the fact 'the qualities that characterize midwifery care, including providing complete information, encouraging self-determination and being sensitive to the emotional state, are particularly important at this time' (Thorstensen 2000).

Undoubtedly funding issues are at play here, particularly in the cash-starved British NHS. Economic pressures combined with the cultural taboos on pregnancy loss, the non-normative mother or 'mother-without-child' (Hansen 1997) is an important 'lost' object. As a focal point of social exclusion and/or intervention, she epitomizes maternal marginality. When she can be judged to be 'deviant' in a sexual as well as reproductive/physical sense, the mother or mothers are additionally excluded.

As we have noticed in our examination of the pregnancy loss literature, silencing and exclusion of the uncomfortable subject of loss is not restricted to the medico-legal 'mainstream'. It is hard to locate pregnancy loss in the lexicon of feminism: Feminists have been well taught to mistrust the concept of the 'pre-born' child, the now-ubiquitous foetal image which threatens to take over the mother's subjectivity and agency (Petchesky 1987). The dangers of 'burying' women's experience is far reaching and damage is done to women's emotional lives, confidence, and sense of self. Because there is so little social and cultural recognition of lost pregnancies, they retain an astonishing power to haunt the potential parents who are enjoined to publicly gloss over the loss of their almost-babies, as Mantel (2003: 228) has described:

> Children are never simply themselves … Their lives start long before birth, long before conception, and if they are aborted or miscarried or simply fail to materialise at all, they become ghosts within our lives. Women who have miscarried know this, of course, but so does any woman who has ever suspected she is pregnant when she wasn't. It's impossible not to calculate, if I had been,

> it would have been born, let's see, in November, ice on the roads, early dark; it would have been the offspring of late March, a child of uncertain sun and squalls.

Pregnancy loss adds another dimension of 'ghostliness' to the abject construction of reproduction and maternity in western societies. (See Layne, this volume.) If the mother remains an 'absent presence' (Kaplan 1992: 3), in the case of loss she conceives another. The lesbian/queer woman is another abiding 'absent presence' in medico-legal regulation and discourse. Just as she is often presumed (wrongly) to be excluded from reproductive life, her experience of loss fails to 'fit' even within the limited cultural outlets for the expression of grief and support, such as web-based support boards. (Though we do not mean to imply that such virtual support communities as www.babyloss.org and www.sands.org are deliberately exclusionary of non-normative sexualities and reproductive contexts, membership and postings are nonetheless dominated by heterosexual couples who have experienced loss.) And the context in which the lesbian woman must 'just try again' is a far more complex and socially fraught than for many heterosexual women.

Concluding Remarks

In concluding, we offer practical suggestions for improving women's experience of early sonographically-detected miscarriage aimed at mitigating some of the negative implications of pregnancy loss. First, health professionals should ensure that: information that ultrasound could reveal pregnancy loss be provided in preparatory materials given to women; and information about what to expect (physically and emotionally) from miscarriage could be provided shortly after the expected loss is identified. Second, health professionals should demonstrate awareness and sensitivity to women's relational contexts and ensure, in the case of lesbian couples, that partners are acknowledged and actively included in consultations. And that for single mothers by choice whether gay or straight, and other women who have used ARTS that awareness of the special difficulty it took to achieve a pregnancy be acknowledged. There is a clear need for improved and broadened practitioner education, but truly sensitive, flexible treatment of pregnancy loss will require wider and less easily achievable cultural shifts in assumptions and expectations about pregnancy, loss and motherhood, and subsequent policy changes.

References

Cooke, K. 2001. *The Rough Guide to Pregnancy and Birth*. London: Rough Guides.

Cosgrove, L. 2004. The aftermath of pregnancy loss: a feminist critique of the literature and implications for treatment. *Women & Therapy*, 27(3-4), 107-122.

Cote-Arsenault, D., Scare, P. and Layne, L.L. (2006) Improving care: reducing the trauma of loss through better preparation and care. [Online]. GMU-TV Programming, Available at: http://gmutvserver.gmu.edu/sdpgen/qt/Motherhood_Lost/subsequent.mov [accessed 2 December 2011].

Davis-Floyd, R. and Dumit, J. (eds) 1998. *Cyborg Babies: From Techno-Sex to Techno-Tots*. New York: Routledge.

Eisenberg, A., Murkow, H.E. and Hathaway, S.E. 1991. *What to Expect When You're Expecting*. New York: Workman Press.

Ellis, C. 2004. *The Ethnographic I: A Methodological Novel about Autoethnography*. Walnut Creek, CA: AltaMira Press.

Ferrara, I., Balet, R. and Grudzinskas, J.G. 2000. Intrauterine insemination in single women and lesbian couples: a comparative study of pregnancy rates. *Human Reproduction*, 15(3), 621-625.

Foucault, M. 1980. *Power/Knowledge: Selected Interviews and Other Writings 1972-1977*. New York: Pantheon.

Foucault, M. 1990. *The History of Sexuality, vol. 1*. London: Penguin.

Golombok, S., Perry, B., Burston, A., Murray, C., Mooney-Somers, J., Stevens, M. and Golding, J. 2003. Children with lesbian parents: a community study. *Developmental Psychology*, 39(1), 20-33.

Griebel, C.P., Halvorsen, J., Golemon, T.B. and Day, A.A. 2005. Management of spontaneous abortion. *American Family Physician*, 72(7), 1243-1250.

Hammonds, C. 2009. My first scan showed up a missed miscarriage. How could I have miscarried without knowing? Available at: http://www.babycentre.co.uk/pregnancy/antenatalhealth/scans/missedmiscarriage/ [accessed 5 December 2011].

Hansen, E.T. 1997. *Mother without Child: Contemporary Fiction and the Crisis of Motherhood*. Berkeley and Los Angeles: University of California Press.

Harpel, T.S. 2008. Fear of the unknown: ultrasound and anxiety about fetal health. *Health*, 12(3), 295-312.

Jauniaux, E., Johns, J. and Burton, G.J. 2005. The role of ultrasound imaging in diagnosing and investigating early pregnancy failure. *Ultrasound in Obstetrics & Gynaecology*, 25(6), 613-624.

Kaplan, E.A. 1992. *Motherhood and Representation: The Mother in Popular Culture and Melodrama*. New York: Routledge.

Kitzinger, C. 1996. The token lesbian chapter, in *Feminist Social Psychologies: International Perspectives*, edited by S. Wilkinson. Buckingham: Open University Press, 119-144.

Kitzinger, S. 2003. *The New Pregnancy and Childbirth: Choices and challenges. 4th Edition.* London: Dorling Kindersley.

Layne, L.L. 2003. *Motherhood Lost: A Feminist Account of Pregnancy Loss in America.* New York: Routledge.

Layne, L.L. 2006. A women's health model for pregnancy loss: a call for a new standard of care. *Feminist Studies*, 32(3), 573-600.

Layne, L.L. 2007. *Designing a woman-centered health care approach to pregnancy loss: lessons from feminist models of childbirth, in Reproductive Disruptions: Gender, Technology*, edited by M. Inhorn. Oxford: Berghahn Books, 79-97.

Layne, L.L. 1992. Of fetuses and angels: fragmentation and integration in narratives of pregnancy loss. Knowledge and Society: *The anthropology of science and technology*, 9, 29-58.

Maclean, S. and Layne, L.L. 2006. Preparing for home pregnancy loss. [Online]. *GMU-TV Programming,* Available at: http://gmutvserver.gmu.edu/sdpgen/qt/Motherhood_Lost/maclean.mov [accessed 2 December 2011].

Mamo, L. 2007. *Queering Reproduction: Achieving Pregnancy in the Age of Technoscience.* Durham: Duke University Press.

Mantel, H. 2003. *Giving up the Ghost: A Memoir.* London: Harper Perennial.

Nanda, K., Peloggia, A., Grimes, D., Lopez, D. and Nanda, G. 2006. Expectant care versus surgical treatment for miscarriage. *Cochrane Database of Systematic Reviews*, 2, 27. [Online]. Available at: http://onlinelibrary.wiley.com/doi/10.1002/14651858.CD003518.pub2/full [accessed 2 December 2011].

Nikcevic, A.V. 2003. Development and evaluation of a miscarriage follow-up clinic. *Journal of Reproductive and Infant Psychology*, 21(3), 207-217.

Peel, E. 2010. Pregnancy loss in lesbian and bisexual women: an online survey of experiences. *Human Reproduction*, 25(3), 721-727.

Petchesky, R. 1987. Foetal images: the power of visual culture in the politics of reproduction. *Feminist Studies*, 13(2), 263-292.

Puddifoot, J.E. and Johnson, M.P. 1997. The legitimacy of grieving: The partners' experience at miscarriage. *Social Science & Medicine*, 1, 837-45.

Renner, C.H., Verdekal, S., Brier, S. and Fallucca, G. 2000. The meaning of miscarriage to others: is it an unrecognized loss? *Journal of Personal & Interpersonal Loss*, 5(1), 65-76.

Royal College of General Practitioners 1997. *Emma's Diary: A Week by Week Guide to Your Pregnancy.* Berkshire: Philip James.

Saffron, L. 2001. It's a Family Affair: *The Complete Lesbian Parenting Book.* London: Diva Books.

Sheach Leith, V.M. 2009. The searching for meaning after pregnancy loss: an autoethnography. *Illness, Crisis & Loss*, 17(3), 201-221.

Smith, L.F., Frost, J., Levitas, R., Bradley, H. and Garcia, J. 2006. Women's experiences of three early miscarriage management options. *British Journal of General Practice*, 56(524), 198-205.

Sotiriadis, A., Makrydimas, G., Papatheodorou, S. and Ioannidis, J.P.A. 2005. Expectant, medical, or surgical management of first-trimester miscarriage: a meta-analysis. *Obstetrics and Gynecology*, 105(5), 1104-1113.

Swain, H. and Layne, L.L. (2005) Enhancing public understanding: normalizing miscarriage through popular culture. [Online]. *GMU-TV Programming.* Available at: http://www.gmutv.gmu.edu/shows/motherhood_lost.asp?ep=11 [accessed 2 December 2011].

Swanson, K.M., Connor, S., Jolley, S.N., Pettinato, M. and Wang, T.J. 2007. Contexts and evolution of women's responses to miscarriage during the first year after loss. *Research in Nursing & Health*, 30(1), 2-16.

Thorstensen, K.A. 2000. Midwifery management of first trimester bleeding and early pregnancy loss. *Journal of Midwifery & Women's Health*, 45(6), 481-497.

Toevs, K. and Brill, S. 2002. *The Essential Guide to Lesbian Conception, Pregnancy, and Birth.* Los Angeles, CA: Alyson.

Ussher, J. 1991. *Women's Madness: Misogyny or Mental Illness?* New York: Harvester Wheatsheaf.

Wieringa-de Waard, M., Ankum, W.M., Bonsel, G.J., Vos, J., Biewenga, P. and Bindels, P.J.E. 2003. The natural course of spontaneous miscarriage: analysis of signs and symptoms in 188 expectantly managed women. *British Journal of General Practice*, 53(494), 704-708.

Wojnar, D. 2007. Miscarriage experiences of lesbian couples. *Journal of Midwifery and Women's Health*, 52(5), 479-485.

Wojnar, D. and Swanson, K.M. 2006. Why shouldn't lesbian women who miscarry receive special consideration? A viewpoint. *Journal of GLBT Family Studies*, 2(1), 1-12.

Chapter 7

Surrogate Losses: Failed Conception and Pregnancy Loss Among American Surrogate Mothers

Zsuzsa Berend

Surrogates talk of pregnancy loss as a painful and traumatic experience even though they emphatically disclaim any attachment to the foetus they carry. Because surrogates feel confident in their ability to provide a child to couples who do not have this capacity, they are especially vulnerable to feelings of 'failure' and loss when their pregnancies fail. But because they are pregnant for someone else, surrogates are denied sympathy at the loss even more than women who are pregnant with their own child (also see Berend 2010). In this chapter I examine discussions on www.surromomonline.com (SMO), one of the largest surrogacy support websites in the world, to document how surrogate mothers make collective sense of what it means to lose a pregnancy that they never intended to be their own.[1]

There are no available statistics of surrogate miscarriages and stillbirths, or on the effects of the extensive medication many surrogates take, on reproductive outcomes or long-term health of surrogates. Given that multiple pregnancy rates are higher among surrogates due to assisted reproductive practices, and that miscarriage is about three times as likely with multiples as with singletons, it is fair to assume that surrogates suffer more frequent pregnancy losses than other pregnant women.

The ways in which surrogates think about gestation, the foetus, and technology are central to understanding surrogacy, including the definition of, as well as the emotional reaction to, loss. In surrogates' narratives, reproductive technology is sacralised; in combination with surrogates' proven fertility, it promises the fulfilment of dreams. 'Medical Technology is amazing, we are so lucky to be in this part of the world where medical miracles happen.' The following consolation, offered to a surrogate who lost triplets, frames technology as sacred when it creates multiples; the negative outcome is understood as a lack of technology. 'Look how much technology went into creating those three little miracles. Why doesn't the technology exist to keep them there? It's completely unfair … ' However, it is their faith in technology, its potential and promise, which leads to feelings of

1 Both Ragone (1994) and Teman (2010) documented that surrogates disclaim attachment to the baby and instead bond with the IP (intended parent).

disappointment, even devastation. But as the above post shows, faith is not lost. In an intriguing shift from faith to fairness, it calls for more technology to produce more miracles as if we were entitled to medical miracles the same way we are entitled to fairness. The meanings surrogates attach to their experience are key to understanding their 'ground of action and stakes of action, with real outcomes in the real world' (Ortner 1997: 10). These outcomes include normalizing and advocating for assisted reproductive technologies, delineating what can be done to whom, and also constructing new models of feelings. It is not simply experts (fertility specialists and clinics) or elites (well-informed and educated intended parents) in the forefront of change. Surrogates exert 'narrative power' (Roberts 1998: 108) as they make collective sense – cognitively, morally and emotionally – of loss in the context of assisted reproduction and thereby enable and establish new patterns of practice.

I found that surrogates experience a wide range of losses, the meanings of which are worked out collectively on SMO. I argue that this forum provides validation and support but also has negative consequences for its members. Determination is applauded and supported on SMO, inspiring women to repeatedly bear children for others even at the cost of their own health. This willingness, in turn, often encourages intended parents (IPs) and medical professionals to push beyond the limits of safe practice.

Using Cyber-ethnography

My data come from SMO, the main online forum for surrogates and 'intended parents.'[2] Founded in 1997 and operated by surrogates, SMO has over 6,000 members (as of August 2011), which has risen from less than 800 when I started tracking it in 2002. The site contains over 1.7 million posts; the overwhelming majority written by American surrogates. Threads get hundreds of 'views' and ten to 25 replies, although some get much more. The more vocal women reach around a thousand posts a year. Combining the characteristics of both written and oral interactions, this online communication interactively builds common experience and shared values; it constructs shared worlds. Debates and arguments can strengthen SMO 'sisterhood;' they give rise to inside jokes that confirm belonging, serve as initiation ritual for 'newbies,' and motivate surrogates and would-be surrogates to reiterate their common purpose.

I chose cyber-ethnography as a research method because the Internet is central to the recent flourishing of American surrogacy. By immersing myself in this online social world I came to understand its language and rules of interaction. Surrogates on SMO talk to one another about intimate matters in a way that establishes a public record. Women assert that while not revealing participants'

2 All quotes are from SMO and online surrogacy journals following links on SMO posts. I use pseudonyms and do not include the URL for my quotes to protect their identity.

identity is important, it is equally important to post 'the good, the bad, and the ugly' so that others may be educated. Surrogates collectively construct what is public by also delineating what is not. 'What we choose to share is up to all of us,' as members can privately e-mail one another through their 'profiles.'

Constructing Loss

Surrogates articulate the meaning of loss as the failure to give a baby to the intended parents. Their anguished accounts are consistent with their oft-repeated claims that they bond with the couple for whom they carry. Their grieving is also an attempt at sharing the IPs' heartache. Surrogates also mourn the loss of the 'journey' and if they are 'first timers' the dream of fully belonging to the surrogate community. Repeat surrogates miss the focus and purpose surrogate pregnancy provides.

What women on SMO call 'loss' includes a range of events or non-events: cancelled 'embryo transfers,' ('embryo transfer' is a procedure where the fertilized eggs are put in a plastic catheter, which is placed near the top of the uterus; the catheter is guided by ultrasound imaging and once in place, the pre-embryos are expelled into the uterus), failed conception, chemical pregnancy, miscarriage, premature labour and stillbirth. The broken heart emoticon () is used not only in posts about miscarriages and stillbirths but also about chemical pregnancies and failed transfers. The following posts by surrogates illustrate this broad range of reproductive loss. 'We had 3 losses … a miscarriage at 6 weeks, 6 days, a chemical pregnancy at 5 weeks, 2 days, and our last miscarriage at 14 weeks, 2 days,' posted Louise. 'It's hard to deal with any loss no matter what gestational age … they were still babies in the dish before they were even put in the womb,' wrote Natalie.

She is by no means alone in seeing 'babies in the dish.' Lea posted 'Pictures of IM's embies!!' Enthusiastic responses from other surrogates and IMs (intended mothers) followed. 'OMG they're beautiful!! Congratulations.' The IM posted too, 'THANKS LEA FOR POSTING A PICTURE OF MY BABIES … COME ON LIL EMBIES GROW. YOUR MOMMY LOVES YOU DEARLY I AM WAITING WITH OPEN ARMS.' After a negative pregnancy test, Lea broke the news on SMO. 'It looks like this transfer failed. We are just shocked… Right now we are just reeling and feeling stunned.' And 'Those embryos looked fabulous. I'm so sorry for your loss,' was a typical sympathetic answer by another surrogate who offered consolation to Lea and her IM. Losses in the heart, then, parallel 'conceptions in the heart' (Ragone 1994).

Then there are losses in the body. Miscarriage is a common experience among surrogates. Nelly lost a pregnancy at ten weeks: 'I could have never imagined the feelings that go along with a miscarriage. Grief, pain, responsibility for this little life …' Liz lost triplets at 18 weeks. 'It was the most horrible, most painful experience ever. … I couldn't give my IP's their miracle … It's going to take some time for me to get over this.'

There are some striking similarities in the narrative accounts of these different types of loss. When surrogates and their couples attempt to jointly make a baby, the boundaries between hope and potential life are blurred. Surrogates' accounts are consistent with the relational approach to the middle-class pregnancy experience Layne (2003) has documented; the primary relationship, however, is not between the surrogate and the foetus or foetuses, but between the surrogate and her couple. Women's relationship to the foetus/es and surrogates' relationship with their couple are informed by many of the same cultural ideas and ideals about the preciousness of children, the importance of family and the emphasis on intent as central to parenthood.

What is specific to surrogacy is the double bind these ideas create for surrogates who experience reproductive loss. Because they consider infertility a major misfortune, they are very sympathetic to childless couples' quest for a baby. When conception or pregnancy does not succeed surrogates feel they let their IPs down. They are sympathetic to the couple's perceived loss and often match the intensity of the couple's perceived sadness, affirming their commitment to a 'shared journey.' Unless the couple is devastated by the loss, the value of the life the surrogate created, and thus the value of her sacrifice is called into question. The preciousness of babies is the foundational idea of SMO.

In her excellent study of pregnancy loss, Layne (2003: 16) argues that women who lose a pregnancy are caught between 'two contradictory sets of powerful cultural forces.' While the first faint positive on a home pregnancy test is increasingly construed as indicative of the beginning of life, pregnancy loss is not considered a death, rather, it is defined as a medical event and women who miscarry are denied full sympathy. The optimistic and voluntaristic climate of middle-class family planning has encouraged women to think of pregnancy as a purposeful undertaking over which they have control; miscarriage shatters this sense of control.

Surrogates' narratives testify to a striking sense of agency and control. 'I have learned that I know my body much better than the doctors. I felt that I could be pregnant successfully again and I was. I wanted to be able to give the gift of parenthood to another couple and I did that.' Even when surrogates talk about fertility and pregnancy as a 'blessing,' they take action to 'share' it with their couple and 'make people's dreams come true.' My contention is that when surrogates claim agency in achieving pregnancy they leave themselves more vulnerable to 'failure' and loss. But because they are pregnant for someone else, surrogates are denied sympathy at the loss even more than women who are pregnant with their own child.

Loss is produced in three distinctive ways. First, reproductive technologies contribute to a sense of loss by holding out the hope of success if people are willing to 'do what it takes' to have a baby. Surrogacy is typically considered the last resort. Egg donors' and surrogates' proven fertility and successful pregnancies seem to guarantee success even if other options failed. Surrogates' expectation of success is thus intimately related to the highly goal-oriented effort the parties engage in. Scholars of assisted reproductive technologies have described the logic:

the more couples keep trying, the more their desire, indeed 'desperation' for a child is confirmed and reproduced; they feel they have no choice but to keep trying. This logic also holds for surrogates. The more they sympathise with their couple, the more they try, and the more desperately they want to 'give' the baby. Surrogates resolutely pursue the dream of helping others: 'This is what I wanted to do, I am such a goal oriented person. I set my mind to it and go for it, I work as hard as I can doing everything I can to reach it,' wrote a surrogate.

Perseverance is routinely met with encouragement partly because the problem is always presented as a heroic tension between IPs' 'normal' desire for a child and their physical inability to have one. This story structure implies that given the availability of reproductive options, joint perseverance is the key to overcoming obstacles. In these stories, not giving up is rewarded in the end. In Western cultures principled purpose and rational pursuit of goals is existentially meaningful and morally good.

The middle-class belief that purposeful effort brings results and it is a moral imperative to finish what you started impacts women's thinking about pregnancy (Layne 2003) and is especially resonant with surrogates. 'I really DO NOT want to give up on surrogacy. I feel it is a calling,' wrote Christine who had been trying to get pregnant for her couple for over a year. Sheryl, whose seven years of surrogacy included two births, one current pregnancy, two early miscarriages and eight failed attempts was supportive: 'Keep the faith … You have not failed as long as you are still trying!' When repeated efforts fail, the feeling of loss is magnified; perseverance contributes to the experience of loss.

Second, assisted reproductive technologies inadvertently assist in the creation of pregnancy loss, especially when they attempt to maximise results. Typically, several pre-embryos are transferred into the surrogate's uterus in order to achieve pregnancy.[3] If they fail to implant and grow, this is experienced as a loss of a potential baby. Transferring multiple pre-embryos increases both expectations of success and the likelihood of multiple pregnancy with its higher chance of miscarriage, stillbirth, complications, even infant death.[4]

Surrogates have many reasons to want multiples. If a baby is a precious gift, multiple babies are an even greater gift. Multiples are a financial gift, too; two or

3 On an SMO poll started in November 2009 over 30 per cent of the 142 respondents answered yes to 'Is it OK to transfer 6 or more embryos?' On a different poll about 'how many embryos did you transfer at a time,' started in February 2009, of the 205 respondents only 9 per cent transferred one, 52 per cent transferred two, 37 per cent transferred three, and 14 per cent transferred five, and over 10 per cent transferred more than five pre-embryos (% exceeds 100 because several respondents did more than one surrogacy).

4 Clinical studies consistently find increased risks associated with multiple pregnancy. For example, one study reported that 'the miscarriage rate for … triplets was 25 per cent, compared with 6.2 per cent for triplets reduced to twins (Yaron et al. 1999: 1268). Twins are five times and triplets are nearly 15 times more likely than singletons to die within a month of birth (see National Vital Statistics Reports (Martin 2005)).

three babies for the price of barely more than one. Even though surrogates do not look for hardship, being pregnant with multiples is genuine sacrifice that transcends 'business.' SMO itself provides another powerful motivation; carrying multiples is usually harder and generates more of a story, thus more interest, support, and praise from fellow surrogates. Although women know that multiple pregnancy is risky, the role of technology in producing loss mostly goes unacknowledged, as in the following post, aimed at consoling a surrogate who lost triplets at eighteen weeks. 'Losing triplets around 20w is EXTREMELY common.' There is no mention, however, that under normal conditions, triplets are extremely uncommon. The rate of natural twin birth is about one per cent, and the triplet rate is about 0.01 per cent. Based on ten years of self-reporting on SMO, twin rates have been between 18 and 27 per cent, while triplet rates around five per cent of the reported surrogate births.

The third way pregnancy loss is produced is via the frequent monitoring and reporting of early positive results (Layne 2012) which stems from surrogates' eagerness to bring good news to the IPs as well as to generate news on SMO. Going through '$100 worth of pregnancy tests' is not unusual. Surrogates post pictures of test results, asking if others also see the faint line. This public wishful thinking contributes to the 'reality' of pregnancy even before the fact; as Layne pointed out, what would have been a 'late period' becomes 'loss.' When the pregnancy is not viable (or not a 'real' pregnancy), surrogates have to 'untell' a whole range of people. If telling establishes the reality of pregnancy; untelling constructs loss.

Anna got positive home pregnancy test results five, seven, and eleven days after the transfer but the official blood tests were negative. She reported that according to the reproductive endocrinologist 'this is a chemical pregnancy. Nothing ever developed far enough to even call it a miscarriage. Not in my books. A baby is a baby no matter how big or small.' Fellow surrogates agreed that this was a miscarriage, and all strongly encouraged her to try again. This thread testifies to the generally shared understanding of what a 'baby' is. It also betrays a tacit prestige ranking of pregnancy-related events among surrogates on SMO where miscarriage counts more than chemical pregnancy which ranks higher than no pregnancy. Pregnancy, even a short one, is more of a surrogacy than no pregnancy; a miscarriage is more of a giving than a failed conception.

Foetal Personhood

In order to understand how the disparate incidents called 'loss' elicit similar emotional reactions, we need to consider surrogates' conceptualization of the personhood of the foetus, and the pre-embryo. The medicalisation of pregnancy and advances in reproductive technologies, together with a range of socio-political developments, has led to a new public elaboration of the personhood of the wished-for child (Layne 2003, Morgan 1998). Surrogates, precisely because they are pregnant for someone else, enthusiastically elaborate the separateness and independent personhood of the foetus.

The foetus-baby is a joint discursive achievement of surrogates and couples. The more intended parents consider the embryo and foetus to be a child, the more surrogates see them as deserving parents. Surrogates and couples also downplay the difference between hope for a child and a child, and technology assists them in seeing 'babies in a dish.' Home pregnancy tests, for example, register chemical changes that are not viable pregnancies. In gestational surrogacy, 'good-looking' fertilized eggs raise hopes of a successful implantation that never actually happens. Or a step before that, 'high-quality' eggs (either the IM's or the donor's) hold out the promise of easy fertilization that does not come to pass. Underlying the 'baby-making' process is the assumption that eggs and embryos are essentially potential babies; the distinction between eggs, embryos, foetuses, and babies is often erased. Even though embryo is defined as the pre-foetal product of conception from implantation through the eighth week of development, surrogates almost always talk about 'embies' when they refer to fertilized ova 'transferred' to the surrogate's womb with the hope of implantation. As a post on SMO announced 'we transferred 2 8-cell embabies!!!' This practical equation of fertilized ova with babies means that any loss is the loss of a potential child.

'It was so sad. I felt such a loss of hope and dreams I had for that specific child,' wrote a surrogate who miscarried. The majority of surrogates contend that 'it is a baby when the embryo implants into the uterine lining,' and 'life begins at conception,' which in the case of gestational surrogacy happens in a dish. Even though these definitions point to a difference between 'life' and 'babies,' surrogates' posts often testify to a blurring of this distinction. Evelyn's post is a good example:

> It is a baby when the embryo implants into the uterine lining … I would say [life begins] at the point of heart beat, but I miscarried before that point and I still feel like there was a lost baby. Sure he or she might not have ever been able to survive outside of the womb, but it was a very much wanted life.

Women on SMO often reiterate that the IPs' intention to become parents is the real origin of the 'wanted' child's existence. 'This child would have never existed if it hadn't been for the love and desire of the IPs;' as Ragoné so memorably put it, these are 'conception in the heart.'

Surrogates echo, if sometimes unwittingly, the pro-life movement's goal of protecting 'the most vulnerable citizens, the unborn' (see The Unborn Children's Civil Rights Act at http://www.rightgrrl.com/1999/s40.html). Surrogates' broad definition of life and their emphasis on nurturing, 'incubating,' and 'babysitting' is consistent with the view of the unborn as vulnerable, needing protection. As Clara explained on a long thread on the topic of terminating a pregnancy because of some abnormality: 'What about the unborn baby's right to choose life? This is just my stance on the matter: I am not anti-choice of the parents, I am pro-life for the unborn who have no voice yet.' Annie summed up a common self-definition: 'I'm pro-life, not anti-choice.'

Women on SMO are somewhat divided on the question of termination in such cases; most oppose abortion but some say that since it is not their baby, it is not their choice, while others maintain that even though it is not their baby, it is their body and their beliefs that are implicated. Termination and selective reduction in case of multiples brings into focus the conflict between respecting the IPs' decision about 'their pregnancy' and surrogates' own stance that all babies are precious. Surrogates increasingly insist that one should only match with IPs who have the same views on these issues. Surrogates find that terminating a much wanted pregnancy is one of the hardest losses.

Surrogate Mourning and the Lack of Support

When their pregnancies fail, surrogates are confronted with lack of support from the medical establishment. Their experience is consistent with findings about the often casual treatment of pregnancy loss by medical professionals. Doctors and nurses 'had no reservations about saying, 'Congratulations! You're pregnant!' when my first two betas came back. Now suddenly I was never pregnant?' Surrogates on SMO establish their own alternative definition. 'Maybe they don't count it as a miscarriage for their 'statistics' but to me, it certainly is the loss of a baby.'

The three-way relationship between surrogate, couple, and foetus also complicates surrogates' emotional reaction to loss. Emotional loss is sometimes aggravated by lack of financial compensation. Whether women receive payment when they miscarry depends on their contract. Ironically, the conscious planning and wholehearted embracement of the pregnancy, thought to be prime conditions for maternal bonding (Klaus and Kennell 1976), are in fact the conditions by which surrogates establish distance between themselves and the foetus they carry.

After the persistent pursuit of pregnancy and the optimism regarding the outcome (based on surrogates' proven fertility and faith in reproductive technology), failure to produce the baby is emotionally crushing. In a letter to the 'dear little embryos,' Dorothy acknowledged that not everyone thinks of multiplying cells as babies, 'but for your mommy and daddy, you were a dream come true.' Another surrogate reports being very hurt by a nurse who disputed her assertion that she had suffered a miscarriage, saying it 'wasn't a miscarriage, just clumps of cells.'

> I was shocked. Maybe to HER it was 'just a clump of cells,' but to me and my IM, it was the loss of two embryos, two potential babies. And yes, we do believe in life at conception. It was a 6 week gestational age – definitely in the medical realm of 'miscarriage.'

The above account evokes the medical definition of miscarriage and simultaneously upholds a specific lay understanding of the beginning of life. Fellow surrogates sympathized. 'It still hurts emotionally, it still hurts physically and a clump of cells or not .. it's still a baby. It's a loss to everyone involved.' 'A loss is a loss no matter when it happens.'

Ragone (1994) argued that surrogates mourn the loss of IPs' attention after birth. In the case of reproductive loss, the loss of attention is accompanied by additional complex feelings. It is not just the loss of the special relationship, but loss of the IPs' trust and appreciation, or fear thereof; loss of the self-image as super fertile and of the 'surrogate journey' they have been dreaming about, and the associated loss, or fear of loss, of one's status in the surrogate community. This community is there for women even, and especially, when IPs are not. The early enthusiastic postings about the 'journey' are met with equally enthusiastic support, launching many months of updates and stories. When the pregnancy does not happen or ends abruptly, would-be surrogates mourn the loss of belonging to the 'club' of 'pregnant ladies.'

Making sense of loss involves an intricate balancing between distancing oneself from the foetus and identifying with the couple's grief. Surrogates empathize with the couple and 'how much they'd been through' and are distraught by their inability to fulfil the promise of a baby. 'This was more devastating news I had to give to another couple who had put all of their hope and faith in my ability to carry their child.' The contention that intended parents suffer more is supported by intended mothers' posts. When Ariel complained that after the failed transfer she barely had contact with her intended mother, an IM explained that 'another neg[ative] is devastating … another piece of our dream is gone, another piece of our heart / our hopes is gone…' Many contend that 'losses in the heart' are harder to bear and are forever. One IM, who already had two children, reminded surrogates: 'this isn't ALL about you … You are having a miscarriage, yes, … it's *miserable.. But ... that* is my baby that died inside your body … I … will spend the rest of my life missing my unborn child … '

Surrogates are caught between two disturbing alternatives. If they identify with their couple's perceived suffering and put their own second, they end up feeling guilty, let down, even used. If, on the other hand, they foreground their own pain, they may appear insensitive and selfish. In one rare example, a surrogate reminded another, 'Keep your chin up and take time to heal yourself. As surrogates … we get wrapped up in the IP's perspectives and tend to overlook the fact that we have just experienced a MISCARRIAGE.'

Often IPs are not as supportive as surrogates would like. Surrogates mostly attribute this lack of support to the IPs' overwhelming sense of grief and often reiterate that IPs who 'have suffered so much already' must be in extreme pain. The advice is to 'give your IPs some time' as they are 'the ones with this dreaded curse and yet again it has been thrown in their face.'

Sue did not need a reminder; she had given her IPs time. They had not contacted her for over a year, 'since the disaster birth/death' of the surro twins. She later found out that this couple moved and changed their e-mail address, too. 'I went through so much physically and emotionally for them to have a family and this is how it all ends … they vanish into the great unknown like a stranger at the grocery store … ' Nina felt very hurt by the couple's behaviour after her miscarriage. 'I have put my body and soul in to this … and what do I get? … stepped on.' Responses recognized Nina's feelings but were quick to point out that the couple's hurt: 'this was their baby, their hope, their future … your IPs have nothing left to look forward to.'

When IPs 'move on' after a failed pregnancy – couples may give up or decide to work with a different surrogate – the surrogate is left in a 'surrogate mourner' situation, with a diffuse obligation to mourn the loss that is not mourned by anyone else. Having made the commitment to creating a precious child, surrogates want to mark the loss in a way that is commensurate with the value of children. When intended parents walk away as if from a failed transaction, they deny the value and magnitude of the surrogate's sacrifice. The relationship with the IPs, imagined as intimate and lasting, is suddenly revealed to be a terminable exchange. This contradicts surrogates' understanding of what surrogacy is so profoundly that they have no choice but to take on the burden of grieving and remembering, as Ruth's story shows. She carried for a single man, which is not unusual:

> Then she died in the womb. When he [biological father] heard, he turned his back. He wanted nothing more to do with me. … He didn't want to BE here for me (or HER), etc. I put everything I had into bringing him a baby…, and he turned his back on me the MINUTE she died. He didn't care she existed, much less that she ceased to exist. That left no one, NO ONE to even so much as CARE that this beautiful little life, this CHILD had ever been conceived. NO ONE left to CARE about her!! I was the only one! From the moment he told me he wouldn't be at the hospital … she became MY child. She was MY responsibility.

More than two years later Ruth was looking for IPs again. Her signature line commemorated this stillbirth: 'Dear Little Angel. Inside me 20w 5d. In my heart forever. 2y 7m 3 w since I said hello and then goodbye.'

If, as Layne argues, pregnancy loss is treated in American culture as a taboo, this is even more the case for surrogates. Ironically, surrogates' assertion that the baby is not theirs and they are simply the 'vessel' leaves them even more bereft of support. Even though husbands and family members tend to be understanding, they often consider the surrogate's grief excessive, given that it was 'not her baby.' Surrogates' grief is not treated with much sympathy by anyone except other surrogates who offer solace on SMO. 'The normal grieving books … the loss of your child books did not apply – there was nothing! … I think if I did not have this site I would go insane!'

'The gift of life' and 'hope for the future' are favourite definitions of surrogacy; failed conception, miscarriage, and stillbirth turn the gift into loss, hope into despair and thus violate all their core beliefs and expectations. Shelly's story of premature birth at 17 weeks poignantly summed up the gulf between expectation and reality:

> I had dreamed of the day M. and S. would become parents. Their faces would light up with the biggest smiles, and tears of joy would roll down their cheeks. Only the reality of Andrew's birth did not hold smiles or laughter, only tears of sadness and the reality of the loss of their beautiful son.

This account is illustrative of surrogates' tendency to foreground the couple's loss and downplay the surrogate's physical pain and risk. Shelly refused to have a D&C because she 'could never disrespect Andrew in such a way' but in her own account she makes her suffering secondary to the trauma of losing one's 'flesh and blood.' She was determined to give birth, even though it could have caused her uterus to rupture, because she could not let go of the surrogate dream; 'I wanted him to be born into his parents loving arms.'

Conclusions

Surrogates are deeply invested in and emotionally attached to the idea of giving. They feel every loss strongly, both as a bodily and an emotional process. The relationship between couple, surrogate, and foetus magnifies loss; failure to conceive or carry a pregnancy to term means failure to deliver the promised gift. When assisted reproductive technology and fertility specialists fail to live up to the expectations they had raised, it is surrogates who have to tell their couple the bad news; most often they feel as if they had betrayed their IPs' trust. The social actions constitutive of reproductive technology, including medical experts', IPs' and surrogates' contributions to its proliferation, are reduced to an act of personal betrayal; an act that can be remedied only by repeated attempts at giving.

Surrogates' SMO discussions normalise this determination to create life even if it entails risks; women collectively allow, even advocate, practices with ramifications for their bodies. These practices, however, have consequences for the life thus created: babies are sometimes born very prematurely with birth defects or chronic illnesses; some undergo repeated surgeries and do not always survive. The unwavering resolve to 'to give the gift of life' and the willingness to take risks while doing so are not only rewarded on SMO but also consequential for how assisted reproduction is practiced, sometimes with devastating consequences for all involved.

References

Berend, Z. 2010. Surrogate Losses: Understandings of Pregnancy Loss and Assisted Reproduction among Surrogate Mothers. *Medical Anthropology Quarterly*, 24(2), 240-262.

Layne, L.L. 2003. *Motherhood Lost*. New York: Routledge.

Layne, L.L. 2012. Why the Home Pregnancy Test Isn't the Feminist Technology it's Cracked up to Be and How to Make it Better, in *Feminist Technology*, edited by L. Layne, S.L. Vostral and K. Boyer. Illinois: University of Illinois Press, 89-118.

Joyce A. Martin, M.P.H.; Brady E. Hamilton, Ph.D.; Paul D. Sutton, Ph.D.; Stephanie J. Ventura, M.A.; Fay Menacker, Dr. P.H.; and Martha L. Munson, M.S.; Martin, J.A., Hamilton, B.E., Sutton, P.D., Ventura, S.J., Menacker, F. and Munson, M.L. 2005. *National Vital Statistics Reports. Births: Final Data for 2003*. [Online]. Available at: http://www.cdc.gov/nchs/data/nvsr/nvsr54/nvsr54_02.pdf, 54(2) [accessed 2 December 2011].

Morgan, L.M. 1998. Ambiguities Lost: Fashioning the Fetus into a Child in Equator and the United States, in *Small Wars: The Cultural Politics of Childhood*, edited by N. Scheper-Hughes and C. Sargent. Berkeley: University of California Press, 58-74.

Ortner, S.B. 1997. Introduction. *Representations*, 0(59), 1-13.

Ragone, H. 1994. *Surrogate Motherhood. Conceptions in the Heart*, Boulder, Co: Westview Press.

Teman, E. 2010. *Birthing a Mother: The Surrogate Body and the Pregnant Self.* Berkeley: The University of California Press.

The Unborn Children's Civil Rights Act. [Online]. Available at: http://www.rightgrrl.com/1999/s40.html [accessed 2 December 2011].

Yaron, Y., Bryant-Greenwood, P.K., Dave, N., Moldenhayer, J.S., Kramer, R, Johnson, P. and Evans, M.I. 1999. Multifetal Pregnancy Reduction of Triplet to Twins: Comparison with Nonreduced Triplets and Twins. *American Journal of Obstetrics and Gynecology*, 180(5), 1268-1271.

Chapter 8
Focusing on Force and Forms in Cameroon: Reproductive Loss Reconsidered

Erica van der Sijpt

Current thinking and theorizing about pregnancy and childbirth often take a linear time frame as a starting point. Dominant biomedical embryological notions trace the development of a fertilized ovum into an embryo and, eventually, a foetus that is believed to be viable at a specific gestational age. Consequently, pregnancies are conceptualized as gradual processes evolving over time and expressible in days, weeks, months and trimesters. This time-based rationale also underlies biomedical definitions of different forms of loss during pregnancy. A miscarriage entails the expulsion of an embryo or developing foetus that is believed to be unviable; the loss of a foetus that would have been able to live outside the womb but dies *in utero* or immediately following delivery is called a stillbirth. When exactly a foetus is considered viable (and thus, when a miscarriage turns into a stillbirth in case of its loss) is understood in terms of gestational time. Most countries have legally established this moment somewhere between 20 and 28 weeks of gestation. Stillbirths during 'late' pregnancy – the exact starting point of which varies again between different national frameworks – form, together with deaths at birth and in the first week afterwards, perinatal deaths. Even if these different definitions lack universally acknowledged demarcations, what holds true for all of them is the persistent effort to distinguish between (more or less mutually exclusive) categories of pregnancy loss on the basis of fixed temporal divisions. Definitions of loss *after* birth are – though less contested – not less time-based; neonatal, infant and child deaths concern the death of live-born babies within the first 28 days, one year and five years of life respectively.

Such temporal assumptions are often taken for granted in discussions about pregnancy and its disruption in both the global reproductive health arena and the social sciences. Within the current international debates on *risks to* and *of* pregnancies in different parts of the world, timing is often critically at stake in the definition of risky reproductive events. There is a strong emphasis on the supposed risks of delivering a baby too early or too late in the gestational process (for example, foetal age as a risk factor), as well as on risks related to pregnancies that are carried too early or too late in a woman's life (i.e. maternal age as a risk factor) or deliveries that proceed too slowly or too quickly (i.e. labouring time itself as a risk factor). Notions of linearity – of the gestational process of a pregnancy, of the ageing process of a woman or of the process of childbirth –

pervade all of these discussions. International programs aiming to reduce the risks of miscarriage, stillbirth, prematurity and infant mortality during women's risky reproductive careers all build upon the biomedically-defined successive stages of pregnancy and loss.

Even if some anthropologists have noted that such time-based constructions of reproduction and risk are highly particular and culture-specific (Bledsoe 2002, Downe and Dykes 2009, McCourt 2009), most of the social scientific studies on reproductive loss distinguish between miscarriage, stillbirth, neonatal and infant death on the basis of these same biomedical definitions. Some limit their interest to one of these categories and aim at an in-depth study of loss at a specific gestational phase (Bansen and Stevens 1992, Gerber-Epstein, Leichtentritt and Benyamini 2009, Letherby 1993). Others *do* consider various categories (such as miscarriages and stillbirths) together. These studies acknowledge that the meanings and effects of early and late pregnancy loss may not be as different as the separate classifications suggest (Njikam Savage 1996, Jones 2001, Chapman 2003, Layne 2003, Earle, Foley, Komaromy and Lloyd 2008). While the distinct categories are thus discarded on the basis of their comparability – in content or consequence – the underlying time-based rationale remains nevertheless unquestioned. The rhetoric of comparability of 'early' and 'late' pregnancy losses maintains the separate terms and the inherent idea of a linear gestational process which can be divided into fixed, successive phases. Alternative interpretations of embryological development are thus left unexplored.

In this chapter, I put this chronological common-sense in context and perspective. I hereby build upon the insights of Caroline Bledsoe (2002), who, by deconstructing the idea that linear time is the essence of fertility, denounces the biomedical time-based distinction between miscarriage and stillbirth. She argues that in non-Western contexts, different forms of pregnancy loss can be distinguished on the basis of other criteria. Drawing upon 15 months of anthropological fieldwork in a village in the East Province of Cameroon, I will explore how women of the local Gbigbil community think and talk about different forms of reproductive loss and how these ideas relate to biomedical time-based distinctions. I will do so by focusing on cultural constructs of foetal development and maternal health in this particular locale, where pregnancy losses and maternal deaths abound. In my 2007 village survey, 60 per cent of the 240 Gbigbil women who had ever been pregnant indicated to have experienced at least one pregnancy loss in their lives. Maternal mortality rates were high as well; although it was difficult to obtain reliable statistics at the local level, the national estimate of 669 deaths per 100,000 births (Barrère 2005), as well as the many stories about women dying during labour and the several 'near-miss' cases I witnessed in the field are indicative of the situation. Such reproductive mishaps are, however, interpreted in terms that have little to do with foetal or maternal age, or with any other fixed, temporal classifications. Rather, physical force and forms appear to be the central focus of concern for my Gbigbil informants.

Filling with Forms and Force: Embryology Explained

When aiming to understand conceptions and meanings of pregnancy loss in a particular locale, it is necessary to first explore the existing explanations of embryology – i.e. *what* people think is actually lost. In eastern Cameroon, understandings of foetal development draw upon a wider framework that places blood at the centre of life. As an indispensible vital substance, blood (*mekil*) is the container of physical force (*ngul*); it enables human beings to grow, act and function. Yet, the amount of force in one's blood is variable over time. While blood is still strong, fresh, and abundant in young people, during life it becomes weaker, dirtier and depleted due to illnesses, heath, physical work and, for women, deliveries and pregnancy losses. The strength of one's blood determines not only personal wellbeing at a particular moment, but is also of crucial importance for the embryological development of one's children.

For, it is the blood of a woman and the blood of a man – whose sperm is considered a mere transformation of his blood – that will 'mix' and form a mass of blood upon conception. This 'loose' substance which is to become a child later on is called *zəng mon* as long as it does not display clear human forms. Once it has developed into something more firm and human-like, the foetus is called a child (*mon*). The exact dividing line between *zəng mon* and *mon* is, however, very fluid. The division is not time-based but rather contingent upon a particular process of growing and 'filling' of the foetus. This process depends on the strength of the blood of both father and mother; foetuses of parents with strong blood develop quickly, while those inheriting weak blood transform themselves more slowly from *zəng mon* into *mon.*

Even when all human features are formed – somewhere between three and five months after conception – the process of growing and filling continues, in order to provide *mon* with force (*ngul*). It is only when a foetus is filled with a certain level of force, that he or she might be viable. Some attain this level after five or six months, others only at seven or eight months, and the very slow ones or twins may even need ten or eleven months. Once viability and life force abound, it is the foetus who decides when a pregnancy comes to term by initiating childbirth with the own force. Therefore, the final point of a 'normal' pregnancy does not depend on a fixed time frame, but varies according to the parents' blood strength and a child's development pace.

Consequently, what is called 'a premature birth' or 'being born before the time' is paradoxically *not* expressible in terms of fixed months or a particular length of gestation. Rather, it indicates a birth that takes place before the necessary development of physical substance and life force has been completed – whenever that might have been. Premature babies are therefore described to be 'not hard yet' (*mon atəka detaa*) or 'not filled yet' (*mon kolonde*). With the pace of 'filling' being variable and contingent on blood force of the parents, newborns can be premature at five, six, seven, eight or even nine months. That it is indeed not time that determines the maturity or prematurity of babies was made clear to me in a discussion with the 29-year-old Charlotte:

> If you give birth at five months and if you have some chance, the child can live. For example, the husband of my aunt was born at five months. When he quarrels with his wife he says, 'Even if I was born at five months, I am more solid than you are. I can hit you and you will fall.' And it is true: he is very strong!
>
> How do you call these children who are born at five months and continue to live?
>
> We call them *mon kolonde.* So the child is not born entirely. Like when you fetch water in a bucket that you haven't filled completely. You can use the word *kolonde* to say that the bucket is not entirely full of water.
>
> From which moment can you call a child 'kolonde'?
>
> From five months. But even at six months it can be *mon kolonde.* And they often tell me that even some children of seven months can still be *mon kolonde.* And yet, other women give birth at six months and their children are fully normal and alive. But at five months, you should be lucky.[1]

Charlotte's first example is insightful: the man's assurance that he is solid and strong is not only a reaction to the perception that children born at five months are 'unfilled', but it also proves that whether a premature baby continues to live or not depends exactly on the amount of *ngul* present at birth. Of all babies born at a certain gestational age, some may live while others die. That is, some have reached a sufficient level of maturity while others are 'born before their time' with too small an amount of force to ensure survival. The irrelevance of fixed time frames as a basis of prematurity and viability was also stressed by the 32-year-old Peggy, who carried a pregnancy of eight months and wondered why her baby waited so long to initiate childbirth. Since she had always given birth around seven months, she assured me that her child must already be 'growing old' in her belly. She reasoned:

> In the hospital they say that a child is premature from seven months onwards. But that is not necessarily the case. I know a woman who always gives birth to perfectly normal children after seven months. In the hospital they also claim that at eight months, the child is dysmature [*dysmaturé*]. That means that it can already be born, it has already everything, but certain organs or functions are not

1 This quote, like all other quotes in this chapter, has been translated from French into English as accurately as possible. Although people speak the local Gbigbil language, most villagers were able to express themselves fluently in French – the regional *lingua franca* in which this research was conducted.

> totally developed. But how can that be? Certainly not all children are dysmature at eight months, since others can be born normally at seven months already.
>
> How would you recognize a baby born at seven months to be normal or premature?
>
> A premature baby doesn't cry with force. Whereas other children can be born at seven months and cry with force. The child is strong as it should be. And the premature baby also has no reflex to suck your breast. He has no force to drink. His jaws are not well developed. It is still very tender.

These Gbigbil conceptions of vital force are at odds with biomedical categories of viability, which take gestational time or birth weight as its exact, independent and measurable indicators. Medical specialists have increasingly come to phrase the uncertain survival chances of premature children in terms of risk calculations that downplay physical strength and bodily fitness in favour of measurable time and weight (Downe and Dykes 2009, Einarsdóttir 2009). In this paradigm, lack of force is only a mere consequence of a premature birth at a fixed time interval rather than its defining characteristic – as it is for Gbigbil people in eastern Cameroon. Even if the latter also portray the 'filling with forms and force' as a linear process, it is not exact time but the variable strength of parents' blood that underlies the gradual creation of a viable human being.

Wasted Pregnancies and Wrong Deliveries: Losses explained

Considering the Gbigbil ideas on embryological development, it is not surprising that their distinctions between different forms of reproductive loss also disregard exact gestational age. Gbigbil women differentiate between the loss of a *pregnancy* where no clear human being is formed and the loss of a *child* presenting human forms. A loss happening at the beginning of a pregnancy which contains only the bloody substance of *zəng mon* is usually depicted as a 'wasted pregnancy' (*abum ia diggela*), a 'leaving pregnancy' (*abum ia vawa*) or a 'falling pregnancy' (*abum ia song*). Once a pregnancy is perceived to contain *mon,* it has become 'hard' and cannot 'fall' anymore. Denotations of loss change accordingly; the expulsion of the foetus is now phrased as the delivery of a dead child. Common expressions relate that 'the child has passed' (*mon ia nul*), 'the child is dead in the belly' (*mon ia wa abum*), 'she gave birth to a child who is dead' (*abiali mon ia wa*) or simply 'the child has died' (*mon awali*). Most of these expressions are also used to denote perinatal and neonatal losses or even infant and child deaths. Since completely formed foetuses are already called 'children', there is no conceptual distinction between *mon* inside and outside the uterus. As such, its decease always concerns the loss of a formed child embodying the potential of life – whether that happens before, during, or after delivery.

Tellingly, biomedical temporal divisions between early and late stillbirth, perinatal death, and early and late neonatal death all dissolve into the Gbigbil use of the word *fausse couche.* Although this French term is formally translated into 'miscarriage' in its biomedical sense and thus meant to be associated with the first few months of gestation, my Gbigbil informants use it as a synonym for *faux accouchement* ('wrong delivery') which can only happen after a *mon* has been created at a later stage of a pregnancy. 'Wrong deliveries' thus encompass all cases of reproductive loss where circumstances make it impossible for a *mon* to live. These circumstances may be related to a fatal 'prematurity' of *mon* – the flipside of the success-stories alluded to above. This is what the 19-year-old Dorine tried to convey during an interview on the meanings of the term *fausse couche* – a notion I encountered in many cases where I, with my time-based assumptions, had not expected it:

> When can you call something a fausse couche?
>
> We talk about a *fausse couche* when you are over time for four or five months for instance. You go to the field and you carry your cassava, plantains and bananas on your head. If you fall with this baggage, you might have a *fausse couche*; the child will leave.
>
> During which phase of a pregnancy can a fausse couche happen?
>
> It doesn't have to do with time. If you should deliver tomorrow, but you have an accident today and your child leaves, we call it a *fausse couche.*
>
> From which month onwards?
>
> It is not dependent on the month. Even if you have a pregnancy of nine or ten months and you fall badly, the child leaves. All this, we call a *fausse couche.*

Despite my insistence to pinpoint a time interval, Dorine's insistence to come back to the example of the accident is insightful; it highlights how all births that happen 'accidentally' – that is, before the appropriate moment of birth which only the foetus knows – are considered 'wrong deliveries' if they end dramatically. 'Wrong deliveries' can occur at all moments in time, precisely because they are not dependent on time in its exact sense. At most, as with prematurity, they represent bad *relative* timing – with the discrepancy between the actual birth and the envisaged birth being too substantial to allow for survival. This contingency of 'wrong deliveries' was also explained by Elianne:

> When I delivered my daughter at eight months and three days, I thought she would be a *fausse couche*, since my first boy had lasted for eleven months! But

> it was a normal delivery. I know now that girls don't take as long as boys do. My son could never have survived a delivery at eight months.

Next to *fausse couches* being related to incomplete internal developments of *mon*, other 'wrong deliveries' might result from outer forces such as witchcraft or illnesses. Many women noted that even a child who is born seemingly healthy but dies within a few hours or days due to external causes, can still be called a *fausse couche*. 'You didn't deliver normally, did you? The child has passed anyway' was their rhetorical answer to my initial confusion. Thus, different losses that carry the biomedical labels of perinatal, early and late neonatal deaths are all called 'wrong deliveries' (*fausse couches*) in French or 'passing children' (*mon ia nul*) in Gbigbil; what counts is that the (developing) *mon* finally 'passed by' – whatever the specific moment and cause of loss.

This is not to say that these losses are not *experienced* differently by mothers. Women indicate a great difference between the loss of a *mon* that is still in the uterus and the decease of a *mon* that one has seen alive upon birth. They express their experiences mostly in terms of visibility of the child's humanness – its forms and force. Thus, the expulsion of *zəng mon* is often minimized since it does not yet show any human features. Likewise, the loss of a *mon* who died 'before its time' is relatively bearable because its dead and forceless body is immediately taken out of sight and buried without much publicity. Yet, the death of a child that was born well-formed and full of force, and that has been cared for and given a name, is heavily regretted and remembered.

Preoccupations with force and forms surface yet in another way: next to *foetal* physicalities, women also focus on their *own* bodily states after 'wasted pregnancies' and 'wrong deliveries'.

Fighting with Force: Losses Lamented

When evaluating the impact of reproductive mishaps, Gbigbil women agree that pregnancy losses always have more severe consequences for their bodily wellbeing than normal deliveries do. Whether happening in the early or later stages of gestation, aborted pregnancies imply a diminution in blood and force that is dramatic as compared to the loss occurring during childbirth. Women distinguish between the loss of *zəng mon* and the loss of *mon* as to the manner in which these vital substances are lost. In case a pregnancy 'falls' in the initial phase of development, what is considered harmful is the abundant loss of blood – not only the blood of which *zəng mon* is constituted, but also the maternal blood that is perceived to surround and nourish it – which causes a *direct* depletion of a body's force reservoir. Charlotte explains:

> In case of an early abortion, the substance of the child is removed from your own body with force! It was stuck to you and now it leaves. You lose a lot

> of blood because you are wounded inside – both before the foetus leaves and afterwards. Some women even faint. They have no blood left. No force in their bodies anymore.

A woman's force is *indirectly* decreased during 'wrong deliveries' that happen after a human-like *mon* has been formed. In these cases, loss of *ngul* becomes inherently related to the decreased force of the baby. For, a child who is delivered 'before its time' does not have the appropriate amount of force to initiate and manage childbirth, gets 'tired' quickly and is likely to die from 'fatigue'. This, in turn, poses increasing demands on the force reservoir of the pregnant woman who should now finalize the 'wrong delivery' with her own strength; without any incentive from the dead foetus, an enormous amount of maternal force is wasted in the process. It happened to the 17-year-old Michelle, who delivered a stillborn son with the help of her mother and a midwife. She says:

> They forced to get the child out, but it was very difficult. Since the child was already dead, he could not get out by himself. So they had to push my belly, so that the child would take the right direction. The midwife inserted her hand and hooked her fingers to pull the child out. At least, that's what people tell me, since I was already … I don't know. I was already tired, I could not even scream anymore. It was not even what they call fatigue huh? I was already dead.

If a woman's reservoir of strength is already depleted due to multiple previous pregnancies or, more devastatingly, their disruptions, the maternal body can become too poor in blood and force to compensate for the lack of foetal force and succumb as a result. Aware of the dangers of weakness in their babies' and their own bodies, women apply several methods to optimize force levels in both. As they consider foetal development a contingent and unknowable, rather than an a-priori fixed, trajectory, women constantly attempt to accelerate the formation and 'force filling' during pregnancy. Through the consumption of nutritious food, different physical activities and regular sexual intercourse with the child's father (whose semen is considered a substantial source of foetal nourishment), they hope to quickly install a level of force that would allow for the child's survival upon expulsion. Towards the end of pregnancy, women also apply remedies to open the 'passage way' during childbirth and prevent a fatal wastage of energy while the foetus 'forces its way out'. The quicker a delivery happens, the more the force reservoirs of mother and child can be spared.

After both successful and – especially – 'wrong' deliveries, Gbigbil women feel the need to replenish their blood and force levels so as to stay 'in form'. For, gradual depletion of the blood reservoir is associated with growing old and weak and thereby becoming less resistant during future reproductive events. Even if they deem it impossible to get back to previous levels of blood volume and strength once a loss has occurred, women deploy several methods to at least partially restore the amount of blood and force in their bodies. They consume green leaves, drink concoctions containing papaya, milk, red wine or mashed tomatoes – supposed substitutes of blood – and search for biomedical injections, which, entering the veins directly, would offer the quickest boost of energy. To be 'in form' is important for Gbigbil women, whose lives are often characterized by a chain of pregnancies – the development and dangers of which are directly related to one's amount of blood and force.

Reproductive Loss Reinterpreted

This phrasing of the development and dangers of pregnancies in terms of blood strength reveals a completely different view on pregnancy, loss, and reproductive risk than the one portrayed in biomedical international discussions. Indeed, foetal age, maternal age, and delivery duration – three important foci of global concern – seem to acquire different meanings and become based on other criteria than linear time in eastern Cameroon. Even if the gradual development of *zəng mon* into *mon* may seem as linear as biomedical embryological models, this process cannot be traced to *fixed* time patterns but is variable and contingent upon the quantity and quality of the parents' blood. Likewise, the physical degeneration that underlies women's ageing process depends not on the passage of years but on the strength of carried foetuses, determining how much blood and force women will waste during deliveries. Finally, what matters in 'wrong' deliveries is not that time is passing but that foetal force and maternal blood are being lost. The crux of reproductive loss thus seems to be the force and forms of mother and (*zəng*) *mon*, which are inherently intertwined – yet in a way that is undefined and by definition unknowable.

This indeterminacy around embryology and maternity leaves room for all sorts of manipulations around pregnancy and loss. Since the boundary between the loss of a 'pregnancy' and the loss of a 'child' is fluid and ambiguous, women can, especially when disruption happens in the beginning of a pregnancy, strategically appoint what is actually lost – mere 'blood' or a 'child'. The fluidity of foetal development thus offers women a rich terrain for negotiating the beginnings and endings of human life (Kaufman and Morgan 2005) through which they can downplay or dramatize their reproductive mishaps within the given circumstances. Gbigbil women may want to downplay a loss if the event triggered suspicions of induced abortion or caused upheaval within the family(-in-law) that threatens a marital future or other personal goals; they may want to dramatize it if the self-depiction as a 'sufferer' is likely to lead to increased attention, care, and favourable options or future imaginations.[2]

Similarly, women negotiate the fate of their own reproductive lives after pregnancy loss through an explicit focus on their physical force and forms; those

2 Likewise, women often strategically adjust their aetiological explanations of pregnancy loss; their ideas on what has *caused* a particular loss may vary along with their specific social situations (Van der Sijpt 2010, Van der Sijpt and Notermans 2010).

who want to postpone childbearing claim to be too low on force or not yet 'in form' after the previous mishap, while those who are eager to conceive again make explicit efforts to replenish their blood reserves. The fluidity of force levels – of both foetus and mother – thus allows for many possible interpretations of and reactions to reproductive loss in eastern Cameroon. Such experiences could not be completely captured if the fixed biomedical framework would be taken as the only valid reference point to study women's reproductive reasoning.

This is of course not to say that Gbigbil women do not know the biomedical framework or use its health services at all. Interestingly, they may resort to biomedical time-based models that seem at odds with Gbigbil embryological notions if these serve their reproductive negotiations and justifications – like when temporal understandings of 'viability' or 'prematurity' are used to strengthen one's downplaying or dramatization of a particular loss. Practically, biomedical services – especially injections – are explicitly sought in the process of replenishment after reproductive mishaps. Exactly because local notions of foetal and maternal health foreground variability, indeterminacy and personal particularity, they – almost paradoxically – allow for the pragmatic inclusion of biomedical categories and care whenever these seem relevant. The medical model then forms just one of the many possible interpretations favoured by a flexible framework focusing on force and forms. Thus, in this eastern Cameroonian village, it is not the biomedical framework that necessarily defines reproductive events, but the other way around: the reproductive events – the social situations and individual stakes around pregnancy loss – define the necessity and relevance of biomedical time-based models for my Gbigbil informants.

References

Bansen, S.S. and Stevens, H.A. 1992. Women's experiences of miscarriage in early pregnancy. *Journal of Nurse-Midwifery*, 37(2), 84-90.

Barrère, B. 2005. Mortalité adulte et mortalité maternelle in *Enquête Démographique et de Santé du Cameroun 2004*, edited by Institut National de la Statistique (INS) et ORC Macro. Calverton, Maryland, USA : INS et ORC Macro, 225-234.

Bledsoe, C. 2002. *Contingent Lives: Fertility, Time and Aging in West Africa*. Chicago: University of Chicago Press.

Chapman, R.R. 2003. Endangering safe motherhood in Mozambique: prenatal care as pregnancy risk. *Social Science & Medicine*, 57(2), 355-74.

Downe, S., and Dykes, F. 2009. Counting time in pregnancy and labour, in *Childbirth, midwifery and concepts of time*, edited by C. McCourt. New York: Berghahn books, 61-83.

Earle, S., Foley, P., Komaromy, C., and Lloyd, C.E. 2008. Conceptualizing reproductive loss: A social sciences perspective. *Human Fertility*, 11(4), 259-62.

Einarsdóttir, J. 2009. Emotional experts: parents' views on end-of-life decisions for preterm infants in Iceland. *Medical Anthropology Quarterly*, 23(1), 34-50.

Gerber-Epstein, P., Leichtentritt, R. and Benyamini, Y. 2009. The experience of miscarriage in first pregnancy: The women's voices. *Death Studies*, 33(1), 1-29.

Jones, L.S. 2001. Hope deferred: theological reflections on reproductive loss (infertility, miscarriage, stillbirth). *Modern Theology*, 17(2), 227-245.

Kaufman, S.R., and Morgan, L.M. 2005. The anthropology of the beginnings and ends of life. *Annual Review of Anthropology*, 34, 317-362.

Layne, L.L. 2003. *Motherhood Lost. A Feminist Account of Pregnancy Loss in America*. New York: Routledge.

Letherby, G. 1993. The meaning of miscarriage. *Women's Studies International Forum*, 16(2), 165-80.

McCourt, C. (ed.) 2009. *Childbirth, Midwifery and Concepts of Time*. New York: Berghahn Books.

Njikam Savage, O.M. 1996. 'Children of the rope' and other aspects of pregnancy loss in Cameroon, in *The anthropology of pregnancy loss: Comparative studies in miscarriage, stillbirth, and neonatal death*, edited by R. Cecil. Oxford: Berg, 95-107.

Van der Sijpt, E. 2010. Marginal matters: Pregnancy-loss as a social event. *Social Science and Medicine*, 71(10), 1773-9.

Van der Sijpt, E. and Notermans, C. 2010. Perils to pregnancies: On social sorrows and strategies surrounding pregnancy loss in Cameroon. *Medical Anthropology Quarterly*, 24(3), 381-98.

Chapter 9
Bereaved Parents: A Contradiction in Terms?

Samantha Murphy

In the 1920s the creation of stillbirth as a legal category in the United Kingdom changed the status of a foetus more than 28 weeks' gestation: from then on it was to be defined as a *baby*. For Armstrong (1986: 216) this meant that medicine had '…mapped out the first year of [infant] life' which began at 28 weeks' gestation and ended when the child turned one year old; the stillborn had, in effect, become a legal infant. In response to developments in neonatal medicine, which have enabled babies to survive at earlier stages of gestation, the boundary between stillbirth and miscarriage was moved to 24 weeks' gestation in 1992 resulting in yet an earlier start for infant life. The recognition of legal status of the fetus as an infant before it is born extends to the legal recognition of motherhood; women whose babies die are entitled to maternity pay, free prescriptions and other welfare benefits in common with women whose babies survive. Drawing on accounts of stillbirth from a doctoral study, I explore how first-time parents define themselves as parents – and ask if the legal status of the stillborn as an infant means they are able to identify as mother and father or is this ambiguous?

Defining and Constructing Parenthood: From Conception to Infancy

Defining the categories of motherhood and fatherhood is not straightforward. Indeed, these categories are often broadly separated into two constituent parts – the biological and the social. Biological parenthood is concerned with the genetic connection between parent and child, while social parenting highlights the performance of the role of mother and father. With the introduction of new reproductive technologies the category of mother may be divided further, for example, into the category of 'genetic mother' after egg donation or surrogacy (Landsman 2000). While motherhood and fatherhood are defined biologically, they remain contested social concepts that are subject to ideological discussion and debate (Woodward 2003) over such things as who should be a mother, at what stage in the life course women and men should become parents and how parenting should be accomplished. Biological parenthood may also be seen as a marker of 'adulthood' (Bailey 1999, Lupton and Barclay 1997) and for men, a major signifier of masculinity (Westwood 1996).

Of particular interest here is the identification of the beginning of parenthood. For both men and women pregnancy may be viewed as a liminal state – conception signals that they are biological parents but, in social terms, they are not yet parents to a separate infant: they are effectively 'parents-in-waiting'. However, the putative social parental identity can be constructed and planned-for as soon as pregnancy is identified. Even before a period is missed, there is scope for parents to identify themselves earlier than ever before (Layne 1992).

With the identity of mothers and fathers being relational to their baby, as his or her incipient identity develops during pregnancy, then it is likely that parental constructions of identity will change to accommodate this. Rothman (1989: 123) maintains that the baby's separation from the mother is a pre-requisite to identity, but she allows that, '… by creating this foetus, this unborn child as a social being, we turn this woman into "its mother" – defining her in terms of the foetus.' By extension, the father is turned into a 'father' and a whole host of kith and kin into grandparents, brothers, and sisters. As Rothman (1989: 59) observes: '[w]e have in every pregnant woman the living proof that individuals do not enter the world as autonomous, atomistic, isolated beings, but begin socially, begin connected.'

Hockey and Draper (2005: 49) note that this procedure has the ability to bring a '… future identity into the present' though before ultrasound scans were routine, Jolly (1976), observed (at a time) that parents conceptualised their unborn child as having 'lived' before birth. For fathers especially, the scan is an important moment as it reinforces their expectant fatherhood (Barbour 1990, Draper 2002) but Sandelowski (1994) argues that it is also one that minimises a mother's relationship to her foetus as this is now is shared with a wider audience. However despite such claims, in their study of fatherhood, Lupton and Barclay (1997: 144) found that those men they interviewed had resigned themselves to bonding after birth, believing that they, '… could develop an emotionally close relationship with their child from early infancy onwards'.

After birth, the roles that men and women play could be interpreted as socially constructed. While claims might be made that these constructions are based on the biological differences between men and women, there is strong evidence to suggest that biology does not necessarily define which parent will be the most nurturing one. For example, drawing on anthropological accounts of tribes in which men were responsible for childcare and women actively rejected it, Oakley (1973), argued that biology did not predispose women to caregiving even though women were expected to take responsibility for children. Indeed, May (2008: 471) writes that contemporary ideas around motherhood are still part of a, '… powerful nuclear family ideology that permeates all of society and is defined and delineated by strong social norms'; motherhood's overriding ethic is the care of children and the role of mother is one that is institutionalised. It is the mother who is entitled to a substantive period of maternity leave following the birth of a child and this cements her role as primary caregiver. Underpinning this is the construction of motherhood as women's 'biological destiny' (Ulrich and Weatherall 2000). Indeed, the representation of motherhood is such that is has an 'instinctive core' and it is, '… still commonly seen as more essentially a part of femininity, not a split from womanhood as fatherhood may sometimes be split from manhood' (Lupton and Barclay 1997: 147).

Fatherhood has been less extensively explored than motherhood. The 'breadwinner' model of fatherhood that accompanies the 'homemaker' model of motherhood first emerged during the industrial revolution (Williams 2008) but, since the 1980s it has moved on from this stereotype. While in the past, women monopolised the nurturing role, concepts of the 'new man' and the 'new father' have emerged – ideas that have attempted to incorporate, '...men within discourses of caring' (Macdonald 1995). Despite this women are conceptualised as being closer to the unborn child than their partners.

In the case of stillbirth, the roles that parents might play after birth are redundant. Parents are faced with a host of unexpected and different decisions to the ones they would have made had the baby lived. Should they see and hold the baby? Should a funeral be held? Should a post mortem take place? Previous research into pregnancy loss has highlighted the importance of memory construction for parents that allows them to bestow an identity on their stillborn baby. The by-products of medical technologies, such as the positive results from home pregnancy testing kits that are sensitive enough to identify pregnancy days after conception, and the pictures from routine ultrasound scans, are used by bereaved parents to reinforce their own identity as parents of their dead child (Layne 1992). The technologies of expectation move to being the technologies of comfort. However, there is a contradiction ahead for bereaved parents. While medical discourse might facilitate parents thinking of their foetus as a baby, the cultural denial of pregnancy loss suggests that, in reality, their unborn child had no status. This means that the, '... death of a baby, especially a miscarriage or stillbirth, is not awarded the significance needed to legitimate mourning' (Rajan and Oakley 1993: 75). It appears that the personhood of the fetus is conditional and should a baby be born dead this personhood is withdrawn by the individuals that constitute the parents' social circle despite the legal recognition of it as an infant and of its mother as its parent. Parenthood is a relative concept in that a mother or father is understood as such in relation to a child. For the parent whose baby does not live and where there is no social role for the parents to play, the identities of mother and father are open to contestation. As Lovell (1983: 760) found when interviewing mothers bereaved by stillbirth and neonatal death: '[F]rom the moment it was discovered that the baby was lost, there was an abrupt cut-off in the identity construction processes ... There was ... a rapid de-construction of her motherhood.'

After an outline of the methods used to research the experiences of bereaved parents, this chapter goes on to consider how parents define themselves once their baby is stillborn.

Researching Stillbirth

The accounts presented here are taken from doctoral research that explored the experience of stillbirth using a symbolic interactionist perspective. This approach to sociology proposes that while people's worlds are constrained by the structures within which they exist, individuals have agency in the way that they understand the world around them; a soft determinism. Thus, the symbolic interactionist is interested in the ways that people understand and construct the social world they inhabit. With this approach in mind, this study sought to explore the experience of stillbirth. It demanded a qualitative approach and thus I conducted in-depth interviews with ten couples who were bereaved by stillbirth. Of these ten couples, five were interviewed jointly with follow-up interviews with five mothers and four fathers; one father withdrew as he did not feel comfortable with being interviewed on his own. The remaining five couples were interviewed jointly with no follow-up interview. A further 12 mothers were interviewed individually as their partners were not willing to take part. This chapter focuses on the interviews with those parents whose first pregnancy ended in a stillbirth; six couples (two of whom were interviewed jointly with individual follow-up interviews while four couples only participated in the joint interviews) and seven mothers.

Interviewees were first invited to recount their experiences and, following this, specific aspects of their bereavement were explored relating particularly to identity. Interviews took place in the participants' own homes and the average length of the joint interview was two and a half hours (the longest being four hours and the shortest one and a half hours). Of the follow-up interviews with fathers, the shortest was ten minutes and the longest 45 minutes and for mothers the length of the interviews was between 30 and 45 minutes. Of the interviews that took place with mothers only, the range was between 45 minutes and three-and-a-half hours, the average length of interview being just under two hours. Approval for the research was given by an NHS local research ethics committee and the University of Surrey. Data were analyzed using grounded theory (Strauss and Corbin 1990) in order to generate codes and concepts that could be shaped into a theoretical framework to explore the gendered experience of stillbirth.

Claiming Parenthood after Loss

The accounts collected from first-time parents suggested that the experience of stillbirth was such that it rendered their status as mothers or fathers problematic (Murphy 2009). Of the first-time mothers interviewed for this project, all were preparing to be the primary care-givers of their children. When talking of their identity as a parent they had difficulty in seeing themselves as mothers but most of them attempted to do so, for example:

> Amy: When I went off for that four weeks [maternity leave], one of the main problems that I was having was that I didn't feel like I should be at work because I felt like I should be at home looking after a baby, but I couldn't do that and I, I wasn't sure who I was anymore. Because I, by rights I *should have been* a mum, um, but because I didn't have a baby, I *didn't feel like* I was a mum. … I *am* a mum, I've had a baby but I've never had the opportunity to be a mum, looking after a baby (*italics mine*).

Amy was not the only mother who made a distinction between biological and social parenthood; mothers would accept the fact of their biological parenthood but the absence of being able to 'do mothering' compromised their social identity. As it would be expected that a mother on maternity leave would be looking after her baby, these feelings had particular ramifications for some women who, while understanding that they were entitled to their full maternity leave, felt fraudulent. In these cases, while legally they were defined as mothers, this recognition did not help them define as such socially. In response to this, several of the mothers returned to work earlier than they might have done otherwise.

Mothers would call on acts performed on their baby in order to aid their self-definition as mother. For example, the rituals around stillbirth that are routine in many maternity units today – the seeing and the holding of the stillborn – is a way in which parenthood could be performed by parents albeit for a very short period of time. Two participants also evoked the act of giving birth (vaginally, as opposed to by caesarean section) as evidence of their motherhood:

> Hannah: I think I felt it was something I wanted to do for him, you know? It was something that I had to do so I was gonna be strong and do it, and that was fine.

> Grace: I would say the one good thing is that they do make you give birth as opposed to doing the caesarean, I would because at least then I did feel afterwards I had done something, I was a mother, I had actually given birth to him.

Of the 13 mothers interviewed, either as a couple or individually, only two rejected any suggestion that they had achieved parenthood at all:

> Maggie: I think you can only be a Mum if you've got a child. You can't be a mother to a dead child.

> SM: At a lot of the Sands groups I've seen people say 'You are a mum'.

> Tanya: Oh, yes, I had all that rubbish. I don't buy into any of that. No, I did actually have experiences of that and it didn't rest with me very well. I just thought it was them trying to put an Elastoplast over the cut, kind of thing. Do you know what I mean? When let's be realistic you're not, are you? You're not!

> I'm not pushing a buggy around, no one's mentioning my birth, my son, nothing, nobody. So how am I a mother? Let's get real.

Maggie and Tanya's definition of motherhood here encompassed both biological and social motherhood but the biological fact of pregnancy and giving birth was not enough for them. 'Proper parenthood' was only achieved when they had gone on to have another baby and it was the subsequent live birth that took them back to where they had expected to be in the first place; hierarchically, parenthood which is both biological *and* social was privileged here over biological parenthood. As this mother, Hannah, said of the birth of her second son, 'Well, you get yourself back to the state where you were intending to be so it puts that status quo right, you know? It doesn't replace [son] but … we're now verified parents, do you know what I mean?'

The data suggest that some parents privilege the social aspect of parenting over the biological one. However, there is an interesting contrast to be made with the literature on adoption revealing that mothers who achieve motherhood socially still do not meet the ideal: ideal motherhood being both biological *and* social (Letherby 1999). Mothers experienced ambiguity in their self-identity; a subject also raised by the fathers in this study.

Due to the literal embodiment of pregnancy, fathers were unable to call on biology in the same way that women might in order to self-identify as a parent. While one man told me that he felt very much like a father in the initial interview, he was far more ambivalent about his identity during the follow-up one. This might have been due to his perception in the joint interview of what his partner expected him to say. However, like mothers, he too expressed the difference between the biological and social aspects of parenthood. For him, 'true' parenthood was something encompassed by the biological and the social:

> Carl: I understand a father's role, um, but, you know, it is kind of a little bit empty I suppose in terms of, you know, you haven't got that, you know, seeing him grow up, expectation. You know, I was in that supermarket today and I, you know, there was, you know, a baby in a, in a little carry cot and I thought, "Well that would probably be how [son] would be now" and you know so you know yes, yes you were a father but not in the, the true sense of the word.

As with some of the mothers interviewed, Carl suggested a hierarchy of fatherhood where 'true' fatherhood is both biological and social. He was not alone in this view, as in common with the mothers, the other fathers who participated were unlikely to fully define themselves as parents due to their awareness of an absence in their lives. While Carl described the loss of active parenting, other men were more likely to refer to something being missing rather than the role of being a parent:

> James: I, I, obviously, I'm aware there should be a baby screaming .... Sometimes I'm really aware there's someone missing. Even though we never had her here and she's never set foot in this house obviously, but I'm aware.

> Harry: Not really. I mean in some respects we did have a baby but you don't feel. You kind of feel like you're missing a baby.

While there had never been a *live* baby, separate from its mother, the men in this study still noticed the baby's absence. This suggested that they were well aware of the difference that fatherhood would make for them and this problematised their status as father. Where fathers were not present for the interview their partners would often sum up what they thought of their partners' attitudes in the following way: I asked, 'Did [husband] feel like a dad, do you think? Amy: No I don't think so. He's never really talked about that, um, but no, I don't think so.'

It cannot be established whether Amy's husband struggled with his identity as a father, however, the accounts suggest that men whose working life carried on much as it did before the pregnancy, had less of a struggle with their identity than their partners. Moreover, while both fathers *and* mothers struggled with self-definition, fathers mostly talked of the loss in a passive way. Although Carl referred to missing the parenting tasks that he might undertake when the child was older, both Harry and James referred to something being 'missing', In contrast, mothers talked of the loss in an active way: they missed performing mothering tasks and of opportunities to express their love for the child. Charlotte, for example, who also had problems conceptualising herself as a mother, had previously emphasised the emotional and physical labour of mothering such as being able to hug and cuddle her baby. Charlotte told me: 'I don't feel like a parent, you know I haven't got the hands on.'

The active/passive divide in women and men's experiences of loss which was suggested by these accounts reflects the roles they would have played after the baby was born, with mothers planning to be the primary caregiver of the child. As such we can argue that the roles that men and women are expected to take after birth mediates the experience of stillbirth.

Identity and the Wider Social Circle

While it was generally unproblematic for parents to define themselves as parents *biologically*, their wider social circle did not always see them as such. Particular days in the calendar might highlight this disjuncture for them:

> SM: Do you think other people saw you as Mum and Dad?

> George: Not really, well, I wouldn't say so, really ....

> Grace: I painted a mug for you, didn't I on Father's Day? And, you know, one of those, you know, paint a mug but instead of doing it on the thing I wrote on the bottom so not everybody would have to see it. Um, but it was sort of, you know, I think I just wrote Happy Father's Day.

The extracts highlight a particular recognition of an ambiguous social identity solved by them hiding any suggestion of fatherhood from other people. It might be assumed that such behaviour would be subject to disapproval on the part of others. This, of course, was a way in which participants tried to understand how others might interpret the situation they found themselves in which implies complicity in the cultural denial of pregnancy loss by the people who were bereaved by it. The parents who were more militant had a different attitude, demonstrated here by Diane's experience:

> Diane: I had a heated discussion with my mother last week about Mother's Day. She asked me to take my grandmother to church and I said 'No', I said 'I can't possibly, you know?' I just said [that] I wanted to forget about Mother's Day right now. I was having a bad day anyway and she got quite upset by that thinking, you know, that I wanted to forget about her being my mother. It didn't occur to her to actually put me in a Mother's Day category.

Diane was keen not only to be recognised as a mother but also that others understood the difficulty that Mother's Day might have for a bereaved mother as it would foreground her loss and produce conflict over parental identity. Unlike some of the other parents, Diane's mother had not seen her stillborn grandchild and this might have impacted on her lack of recognition of Diane as a mother. Attendant to this lack of recognition of Diane's motherhood was an implicit lack of recognition of Diane's son. Denying Diane motherhood meant denying her grandson existence. This suggests that Diane's mother did not understand herself as the stillborn's grandmother even though she was positioned as such before the birth and Diane related how 'excited' she was: the 'grandson-hood' of the stillborn was conditional on being born alive.

This lack of recognition of parental identity can have wider institutional consequences. As already noted some women mentioned returning to work before they were ready and before their entitlement to full maternity pay ended. These mothers had constructed their maternity leave as instrumental; without a baby to mother there was no need to stay at home as there was no role to perform. For one mother, however, it was obvious that her employers thought that without a baby she was not entitled to the benefits the firm offered and would have been enjoyed had her son been born alive. Grace worked at a well-known firm of accountants which, at the time, encouraged new mothers to go back to work after having their babies in the form of a 'back-to-work' bonus that amounted to 15 per cent of the mother's annual salary and was intended for childcare costs.

> Grace: So I said, 'I get my maternity, return to work?' 'No, you don't, you don't get a return to work bonus, a maternity return to work bonus', and I said, 'Why?' Because your baby's died and, um, it's supposed to, it's there to get people to come back to work when they've had a baby to cover their, um, nursery costs.

Notwithstanding the fact that Grace might well have decided not to return to work, her employer, too, had seen the bonus merely in an instrumental light. While she could see the logic of the firm's reaction, she fought for the bonus and won. The end result, however, was that the firm rewrote the policy resulting in further guilt that centred around the implications her actions might have for other women in a similar situation. While giving birth to a dead baby is financially less expensive than a live one, there is a symbolic message given out here by the firm; that the stillborn is less worthy than the live born.

Bereaved Parents: A Contradiction in Terms?

Theoretical approaches to identity highlight the importance of the roles played by each individual. Before an individual is born, he or she is given a place within its parent's social circle but, despite this idea that the fetus is a social entity, after a stillbirth, it seems it is not. There is, then, an apparent contradiction between the conceptualisation of the baby before and after birth that impacts upon parents bereaved by stillbirth. If the baby was a child that was talked about and included in a family before birth, why is it difficult to do so after death? The personhood bestowed on the unborn baby is, therefore conditional on a live birth leaving the parents in an ambiguous position after death. Parenthood, once seen as assured, has been lost; the stillbirth has emphasised the disjuncture between biological and social parenthood.

This ambiguity over the personhood of the stillborn impacts upon the parents' identity as mothers and fathers – how should they define themselves? Do they have children or not? Indeed, the parents bereaved of their second or subsequent child, that latter question is similar – how many children do they have or, at the least, admit to? The term 'bereaved parent', as applied to first-time parents who have had stillborn babies, is something of a contradiction in terms. If there is no social identity for the baby, then the mother and father cannot be a parent. If they are not a parent, they cannot be bereaved even if some social parenting tasks towards the baby have taken place, that is: the bathing and dressing of the stillborn baby.

In pregnancy the mother is positioned as physically closer to her baby and this closeness is reinforced by the social expectations of the pregnant woman and the role that she will undertake after birth. The accounts presented here demonstrate that both first-time mothers and fathers had difficulty in defining themselves as parents following stillbirth. Thus, there is likely to be a consequential effect on the continued experience of bereavement and, moreover, this effect is likely to be gendered. Women are positioned as closer to the unborn child than men due to the physical embodiment of pregnancy but the gendered construction of parenting also plays its part. Socially, motherhood is seen as more integral to femininity than fatherhood is to masculinity. The expectation that the mother will be the main carer, reinforced by differing entitlements to leave following the birth of a child, all impact on the experience of stillbirth making the loss experientially different for women and men.

To conclude, Jenkins (1996) argued that it is at birth that individuals become social but it seems to me that it can be argued that before birth the parents of the unborn are not merely biological parents but social ones as well. While we might accept Jenkins's position that the unborn infant is not a social being, it is a being that parents are performing tasks towards. The refusal of a glass of wine, decorating the nursery, giving up smoking and naming babies are inherently social acts. Thus, before birth, the baby's social identity may be accepted by its parents and, as the data show, their wider social circle. Accepting the identity of an unborn baby as both social and biological before birth, and accepting that it is actively parented before birth, might be a way in which mothers and fathers bereaved by stillbirth can define themselves as parents. This might be preferable to the ambiguous position that stillbirth leaves them in and which can only be relieved by the birth of a subsequent child if this occurs.

References

Armstrong, D. 1986. The invention of infant mortality. *Sociology of Health and Illness*, 8(3), 211-232.

Bailey, L. 1999. Refracted selves? A Study of Changes in Self-Identity in the Transition to Motherhood. *Sociology*, 33(2), 335-352.

Barbour, R.S. 1990. Fathers: The emergence of a new consumer group, in *The Politics of Maternity Care: Services for Childbearing Women in Twentieth Century Britain*, edited by J. Garcia, R. Kilpatrick and M. Richards. Oxford: Oxford University Press, 202-216.

Draper, J. 2002. It was a real good show: The ultrasound scan, fathers and the power of visual knowledge. *Sociology of Health and Illness*, 24(6), 771-795.

Hockey, J. and Draper, J. 2005. Beyond the womb and the tomb: Identity, (dis) embodiment and the life course. *Body and Society*, 11(2), 41-57.

Jenkins, R. 1996. *Social Identity.* London: Routledge.

Jolly, H. 1976. Family reactions to stillbirth. *Proceedings of the Royal Society of Medicine*, 69(11), 835-837.

Landsman, G. 2000. 'Real Motherhood', Class, and Children with Disabilities, in *Ideologies and Technologies of Motherhood: Race Class Sexuality Nationalism*, edited by H. Ragone and F.W. Twine. London: Routledge, 169-190.

Layne, L.L. 1992. Of fetuses and angels: Fragmentation and integration in narratives of pregnancy loss. *Knowledge and Society: The Anthropology of Science and Technology*, 9, 29-58.

Letherby, G. 1999. Other than mother and mothers as others: the experience of motherhood and non-motherhood in relation to 'infertility' and 'involuntary childlessness'. *Women's Studies International Forum*, 22(3), 359-372.

Lovell, A. 1983. Some questions of identity: Late miscarriage, stillbirth and neonatal loss. *Social Science and Medicine*, 17(11), 755-61.

Lupton, D. and Barclay, L. 1997. *Constructing Fatherhood: Discourses and Experiences*. London: Sage.

Macdonald, M. 1995. *Representing Women: Myths of Femininity in the Popular Media*. London: Edward Arnold.

May, V. 2008. On being a 'good' mother: The moral presentation of self in written life stories. *Sociology*, 42(3), 470-486.

Murphy, S.L. 2009. *Parenting the Stillborn: Gender, Identity and Bereavement*. Unpublished PhD thesis: University of Surrey.

Oakley, A. 1973. *Sex, Gender and Society*. Aldershot: Arena.

Rajan, L. and Oakley, A. 1993. No pills for heartache: The importance of social support for women who suffer pregnancy loss. *Journal of Reproductive and Infant Psychology*, 11(2), 75-87.

Rothman, B.K. 1989. *Recreating Motherhood*. W.W. Norton: New York.

Sandelowski, M. 1994. Separate, but less unequal: fetal ultrasonography and the transformation of expectant motherhood/fatherhood. *Gender and Society*, 8(2), 230-245.

Strauss, A. and Corbin, J. 1990. *Basics of Qualitative Research*. London: Sage.

Ulrich, M. and Weatherall, A. 2000. Motherhood and infertility: Viewing motherhood through the lens of infertility. *Feminism and Psychology*, 10(30), 323-336.

Westwood, S. 1996. 'Feckless fathers': Masculinities and the British state, in *Understanding Masculinities*, edited by M. Mac an Ghail. Buckingham: Open University Press.

Williams, S. 2008. What is fatherhood? Searching for the reflexive father. *Sociology*, 42(3), 487-502.

Woodward, K. 2003. Representations of motherhood, in *Gender, Identity and Reproduction: Social Perspectives*, edited by S. Earle and G. Letherby. Basingstoke: Palgrave Macmillan, 18-32.

Chapter 10
'Troubling the Normal': 'Angel Babies' and the Canny/Uncanny Nexus

Linda L. Layne

Ethnographic accounts of the new kinship practices that emerged in the last few decades with the help of assisted reproductive technologies frequently used the concepts of 'normalization' and 'naturalization' to explain how 'pioneers' of these new family forms dealt with their novel experiences. For instance, Ragoné (1994: 3) describes the surrogate mother programs in the U.S. she studied as 'engage[ing] in a process of normalizing the surrogate mother experience for both their couples and their surrogates' and Thompson (2005: 80) used the concept of 'normalization' to describe 'the ways by which new patients, new scientific knowledge, new staff members, new instruments, new administrative constraints are incorporated into preexisting procedures and objects' of the IVF clinic in California she studied. Franklin noted the prominence of 'nature' in the literature provided by the British IVF clinics and drug companies and how 'nature' was used to 'shift the focus away from the anomalous quality of' this form of family building (1997: 103, 127). The final chapter of Lewin's book on lesbian mothers, titled *Natural Achievements*, describes the extent to which lesbian mothers used 'symbols of conventional (read 'natural') family life … to back up their claims that families headed by lesbian or gay parents, are in fact, families like any others' (1993: 188).

Long-term ethnographic research with a number of pregnancy and infant loss support organizations in US (1986–2010) provides material with which to reassess the adequacy of the concepts of 'normalization' and 'naturalization.' This is part of a larger project on emerging family forms, including single mothers by choice and two-mom families in which I have identified uncanny similarities in the ways that people engaging in these family forms deal with the absent presence of one member of the still normative nuclear family. I argue that while many of the ways support group members construct their wished-for baby as a family member can be understood as acts of 'normalization' and/or 'naturalization,' these concepts do not do justice to the complexity of their family-making practices. Indeed, the 'angel babies' which populate the pregnancy loss support movement are apt examples of 'troubling the normal' (Mamo 2007: 6). One of the limits of the twin notions of 'normalization' and 'naturalization' is that they describe a unidirectional process. The movement is always from the 'socially defiant' to the 'socially accepted' – from 'abnormal' or 'unnatural' to 'normal' and 'natural.' In contrast, the closely related concepts of the 'canny' and 'uncanny,' point to the fluidness of such distinctions and the fact that at least some of these parents' practices move in both directions. Sometimes they make the strange more familiar; other times, their practices, including those of 'poetic license,' accentuate the strangeness of their experiences rather than normalizing them.

The Canny/Uncanny and Poetic License

In a 1919 essay on 'The Uncanny,' Freud gathered together the preceding aesthetic and literary theories on this topic. I draw on Freud's presentation and reflections on these theories rather than his particular contributions to the subject to explore the feelings expressed in narrative accounts. In other words, I am not engaging in or advocating a psychoanalytic approach, but rather bringing to bear neglected aesthetic concepts to discourse analysis in the anthropology of reproduction.

One of the most striking features of the concept 'canny,' *heimlich*, is that it has two nearly opposing meanings. The first is 'belonging to the house or the family … familiar tame, intimate … arousing a sense of peaceful pleasure and security' as within the four walls of one's own house (Freud 1949: 371-2). The second is 'concealed, kept from sight,' that which is 'hidden, secret, mysterious' (1949: 129). It is in this sense that 'canny' resembles its opposite, 'the uncanny,' *unheimlich*, which refers to the 'unhomey, unfamiliar, untame, uncomfortable, eerie, weird' (Freud 1991: 375).

According to one view, 'the essential condition' for creating a 'sense of uncanniness' is 'intellectual uncertainty.' Hence, 'the uncanny would always be an area in which a person was unsure of his way around' (Freud 2003: 125). This sense of the 'uncanny' is also evident from its etymological root. 'Canny,' from the Anglo-Saxon root 'ken,' means 'knowledge, understanding, or cognizance.' 'Uncanny,' thus is 'an idea beyond one's ken,' something outside one's familiar knowledge or perceptions. In the U.S., losing a wished-for pregnancy by miscarriage or stillbirth takes one 'beyond one's ken,' venturing into unfamiliar territory. Freud uses 'the uncanny' to describe 'the class of frightening things that leads us back to what is known and familiar' (Freud nd: 1). Bereaved parents engage in a number of practices that traffic back and forth between the familiar and the bizarre, the comfortable and the strange.

Another helpful concept for understanding these practices is 'poetic license.' Freud refers to 'poetic license' in his essay on 'the uncanny,' noting that this allows 'the imaginative writer' to 'select his (sic) world of representation so that it either coincides with the realities we are familiar with or departs from them in what particulars he (sic) pleases' (2003: 156). In fairy tales, for instance, the world of reality is left behind from the very start, and the animistic system of beliefs is frankly adopted. 'Wish-fulfillments, secret powers, omnipotence of thoughts, animation of inanimate objects'(2003: 156), all common features of fairy tales, are evident in the narratives of these non-normative family-makers. The theoretical concepts of 'the canny,' 'the uncanny,' and 'poetic license' help explain both why participants engage in these acts and why others may judge their practices to be bizarre.

Angel Babies – An Absent Presence

Though pregnancy losses can be understood to be both 'natural' and 'normal,' they are rarely experienced as such, but rather as counter to the order of things, as an aberration (Douglas 1966). Parents who suffer a pregnancy loss sometimes liken themselves and/or their loss to freaks of nature (Layne 1996). Dead fetuses or newborns are liminal and as such have the potential for great power and danger (Douglas 1966). In the U.S., the dangerous valence of these beings is predominant, and like other entities which do not fit into our cultural scheme, they are hidden and ignored (see Komaromy, this volume).

In the wake of the post-1960's uprising of stigmatized groups (Layne 2006a), bereaved parents have been fighting the negative social judgments associated with 'failed pregnancies.' One of the ways they have done so is by adopting the valorizing trope of 'angel babies.' Angel babies have become pervasive in the pregnancy loss support movement; they are evident in the names of several organizations, e.g., The Angel Names Association, Angel Whispers, Still Angels and the Missing Angels Foundation, and routinely found in the poems and first-person accounts published in support group newsletters (Layne 2003). Even in more mainstream popular culture this usage is appearing. For example, the 'Just Mommies' website for 'moms and moms to be' has a page devoted to 'Angel Baby Remembrance' on which visitors describe what they have done to commemorate their miscarriages and stillbirths.

While construing their longed-for children as 'angel babies' valorizes bereaved parents' experience, it does so in a way that brings us into the realm of the 'uncanny.' According to Freud, one condition which is likely to arouse an especially strong sense of the uncanny is when there is confusion between the animate and inanimate, either because there is 'doubt as to whether an apparently animate object really is alive, and conversely, whether a lifeless object might not perhaps be animate' (Jentsch quoted in Freud 2003: 135).

Angel babies are conjured, animated, and domesticated in a number of ways, including sexing, naming, clothing, picturing, treating as imaginary correspondents, as conversation partners, and/or companions, and purchasing consumer goods that serve as a surrogate for the child including life-like memorial dolls.

Sexing and Naming

Most pregnancy losses occur during the first trimester, at a stage during which a number of the prerequisites of personhood may be missing. Most pregnancy losses occur before sexual organs are formed and this makes naming difficult (Layne 2006b). The largest support organization, SHARE, encourages bereaved parents to 'name their baby … whether or not the gender is known' suggest that 'if he/she was lost early, use a name that is gender-neutral' (1999: 5). Another way some solve this problem by intuiting the sex (Allen and Marks 1993: 37). Others feel parenthood gives them the prerogative of choosing the sex. For example, after having two early (6 week) miscarriages, Sandy Smith (1999) 'decided to choose names for my babies. Since I was their mom, I decided to choose their gender.'

Using the baby's name in conversation, on consumer goods, at family and support group rituals is one of the most common ways the baby is purposely made present (Layne 2006b).

Clothing

Another important means for constructing the personhood of a longed-for baby is clothing. Making, purchasing, and giving clothes is a common way that the personhood of an embryo or fetus is socially constructed by the parents and members of their social network while *in utero* (Layne 2000a, b, 2001). In a departure from the past when dead babies were whisked away in an effort to spare the mother, families are now encouraged to spend time bathing, dressing, and holding their dead baby. 'Threads of Remembrance' is a hospital-based organization that provides clothing for premies and micropremies who are born dead. Nurses and grief counselors praise this clothing because it 'offers families comfort, and brief moment of normalcy' (www.meriter.com/content/?cm_id=357 Accessed June 7, 2011).

SHARE suggests parents take pictures of their baby wearing a variety of outfits (SHARE 2010a). Although the reason given for this is 'to add variety to your photos,' doing so effectively creates the impression of the passage of time, i.e., the fiction that s/he lived over a period of time. In other words, this practice is a 'confabulation,' a staging of imaginary events 'to fill in gaps in memory' (Hirstein 2006: 2).

Picturing

Taking, preserving, and displaying pictures of their dead babies is another important way that the babies' presence can be maintained in spite of their absence. Having hospital staff take snapshots of the baby for the parents has become a standard of care in the U.S., and is one of the items listed on SHARE's 'Bill of Rights for Parents whose Baby has Died' (1991). SHARE suggests about twenty poses (e.g., on tummy *as if* sleeping, with mouth open and closed, dressed and undressed…) (emphasis added, www.nationalshare.org/lifetime-memories.html). In a growing number of communities, professional photographers volunteer to go to hospitals to take studio-quality photos of dead or dying babies, thanks to the parent-founded organization, 'Now I Lay Me Down to Sleep' (http: //www.nowilaymedowntosleep.org/stories/).

'Poetic license' is not only evident in the name of this organization but also in their common practice of 'retouching' the photos to 'edit away the bruises, sloughed skin and other evidence of physical trauma' (Ohlson 2010). Bereaved parents feel this fiction is needed in order for them to be able to show the photos to others. Cheryl Haggard, the founder, explains that because the photographer 'was able to digitally erase the trauma of [her son's] short life,' we can share his image with others. '"I don't want pity when I show his picture to people … I want them to say, 'Wow, he was beautiful'" (Ohlson 2010). One of the reasons she and her husband had requested a photographer was so they could have a photograph to hang in their home amid their other children's portraits. Wendy deLong had the same motivation when, eighteen years after the death of her son, she had 'the few pictures' she had of Jarrod retouched. She explains 'You see … he was hooked up to all the tubes and such, and we couldn't really see his face.' She had wanted to have this done for some time but had 'felt a little funny going to a photographer with these kind of photos. I worried a lot about what people would think of me, which I know now doesn't really matter.' She was so happy to have the retouched photos though because 'Jarrod now sits in a frame with both his brother and sister on our entertainment center' (deLoge 2010). The location of these dead babies and the photos of them, on the boundary between the private and public realms, between the 'normal' and the 'abnormal,' at once 'canny' and 'uncanny,' is evident in the fact that deLoge felt 'a little funny' about going to a photographer (an outsider) with 'this kind of photo.' Once retouched, she displayed it in a semipublic space within the privacy of her own home.

Others go further in crossing the boundary between private and public with these 'uncanny' images by wearing pictures of their longed-for baby as, for example, the dad at a MISS Foundation conference who wore a t-shirt emblazoned with a large photograph of his daughter framed by her name and birth and death dates. By making seen what is socially-expected to remain unseen, they defiantly assert their non-normative parenthood.[1] Others inscribe these images directly on their body, either temporarily with henna, or permanently with tattoos.

Angel babies are a popular motif in memorial tattoos, with angel wings affixed to the baby's image or to her/his name. For instance, one contributor to the 'just mommies forum on recurrent miscarriage' had the names of her 'three living kids and [2] second trimester losses' tattooed on her arms. She explained, 'the angel babies are the ones with wings' (http: //www.justmommies.com/forums/f256-recurrent-miscarriage-and-pregnancy-loss/1816022-angel-baby-remembrance.html).

Such a permanent melding of the two bodies (living parent/dead child) is a dramatic means of making the absent family member present, always. One contributor to the baby-gaga website explained that she has been thinking of

1 This assertion of non-normative parenthood is similar to the African American and Latina teen mothers studied by Lustig (2004) who 'prominently displayed' studio photographs of their babies on their persons to proudly and defiantly 'signal their identity as mothers' in a social setting that 'tried to keep the babies invisible.'

'getting Zachary's foot prints on the top of my feet to represent that he walks with me always …' (http://forum.baby-gaga.com/about281287-1.html).

'Poetic license' is also evident in the practice of making the missing family member present in family photographs through the use of surrogate consumer goods. The baby's absence is often felt acutely during family rituals, including the taking of family portraits, and on these occasions, some bereaved parents conjure their missing baby's presence via a symbolic object that acts as a stand-in. One family uses 'a special teddy bear' (Schneider 1996: 7); another has each family member wear a 'guardian angel pin' with the baby's birthstone (Jones 1992). One woman took a picture of her two surviving sons under the memorial tree her husband had given her the first Mother's Day after Max was stillborn. She gave the picture to her husband for Father's Day, 'so that he would see all of his boys, including Max' (2010). It would be incorrect to interpret these acts as acts of normalization or alternatively, as 'wish fulfillment,' however (Freud 2003: 156). As the grandmother of the child represented by the Teddy Bear makes clear: 'Grief is … taking a family picture with Alexander's teddy bear instead of with Alexander' (Schneider 1996: 7).

Conversing and Corresponding With

SHARE advises parents who are able to spend time with their dead baby in the hospital to 'speak to your baby. Tell him or her how you feel' (SHARE 2010a, www.nationalshare.org/lifetime-memories.html, accessed July 16, 2010). Afterwards, many continue to address their babies through letters or poems. Sometimes, they tell the baby that s/he is missed, loved, and still remembered. Other times, 'angel babies' are asked to help their world-bound families (Layne 2004).

Another method for communicating with 'angel babies' is via helium balloons, often released on the baby/ies' 'angelversary'(Fiorello 2010). One mother tells of how each year on the birthday of her 'two angel babies,' she, her husband, and daughter each release a balloon on which 'they have written a message and sing happy birthday to her as they rise.' She also 'takes time to write them letters or make a card, just to feel close to them' (Anonymous). Blowing soap bubbles, like those distributed by the Angel Names Association at their annual walk, serves a similar symbolic function.

Some bereaved parents also experience communication to flow in the other direction – from the angel baby to her/his family via signs. Such occurrences are referred in the SHARE literature as evidence of 'angelic presence.' A special issue of their newsletter is devoted to documenting such experiences and a book of essays on pregnancy loss has that as its title (Lammert and Friedeck 1997). These signs often take the form of mundane natural occurrences, the timing of and location of which (and other particularities such as color and number), are understood to have special meaning. Examples include a cardinal from the sky/heaven that lands on their baby's grave, or a single pink flower that grows in an unusual spot and isn't noticed till the moment that she is opening the envelope that contains photographs of her daughter, or a single yellow tulip growing spontaneously in the back yard after they planted yellow tulips on their baby's grave. Each of these is interpreted as 'a sign of love from' their babies. For example, whenever the one family sees a cardinal, 'our angel redbird,' they know that 'she is close by, watching over us.' These occurrences are comparable to coincidental circumstances Freud describes, that 'transform what would otherwise seem quite [ordinary] into something uncanny and forces us to entertain the idea of the fateful … when we should normally speak of 'chance' (Freud 2003: 144). The 'uncanny,' thus leads us 'back to the … animistic view of the universe,. characterized by the idea that the world [is] peopled with human spirits' (Freud 2003: 145).

Baby Dolls as Tangible Presences

Some make their missing baby present by having a life-like doll crafted in their baby's image. One purveyor of these memorial dolls is a born-again, pro-life, elementary school teacher from Elmira NY, who began sculpting them in 1993, following a miscarriage (http: //godslittleones.homestead.com/artistbio.html Accessed April 2011). The sculpture of an 8-week gestation embryo, pictured on her website in a thimble, was 'made in memory' of her own 'daughter' whom she named 'Amazing Grace.' Her goal is to help parents who have lost a baby through miscarriage, stillbirth, and abortion to 'value them as 'God's Little Ones'.' She hopes her dolls 'bring comfort to many and prove that the unborn are human beings deserving love and respect.' She uses obstetrical charts and scientific measurements as well as photographs of real babies born at each week of development… to ensure the accuracy of each model.'

Another maker of memorial baby dolls is Jennifer Stocks. She started sculpting them in 2006 after her 16-month old daughter died of SIDS. Nearly 80% of the 898 dolls she has created since have been 'memorial pieces.' She uses her mastery of 'the art of "likeness" to create portrait pieces for families who have lost children in pregnancy, birth, to SIDS, or other illnesses … If a family has provided a photograph, I'll do my best to capture as many features and likeness as I can' (Seven Days 2007). One mother who lost a son to SIDS explains, 'I chose Jenn because of [her] remarkable … ability to bring her babies to life' (www.tangiblepeace.org Accessed June 2011).

While the bereaved parents who commission her work find the dolls a great comfort when they look at or hold them, others, including some other bereaved parents, find them unsettling. One observer describes them as 'eerily realistic' (Thompson 2007). Dearborn is acutely aware of the borderland between canny/uncanny that her dolls occupy. On the one hand, her work has provided her a 'tangible peace' and yet she also recognizes that her dolls are 'creepy naked babies.'

There are several elements of the dolls which evoke creepiness. As Freud noted, dolls have a special capacity for provoking feelings of 'uncanniness' because of and to the extent to which these inanimate objects 'appear to be alive.' 'A particularly favourable condition for awakening uncanny sensations is … when an inanimate object becomes too much like an animate one' (Freud 1949: 385). In addition to their life-likeness, the fact that these dolls represent dead bodies adds to their strangeness. As Freud notes, 'for many people the acme of the uncanny is represented by anything to do with death, dead bodies' (Freud 2003: 148). A third element in the creepiness equation is that many of the dolls depict embryos or fetuses, which, when alive, occupy 'secret places [of] the human body' (Freud 2003: 133). Freud notes that this usage of canny is one which overlaps with 'the uncanny.' He uses this meaning when referring to women's pudenda and later refers to 'the fantasy of living in the womb' (2003: 150) (and the related fantasy of being buried alive), as a 'the crown of the uncanny' (2003: 150). He concludes that though 'some neurotic men' find female genitals 'uncanny … what they find uncanny ['unhomely'] is actually the entrance to man's old 'home', the place where everyone once lived' (2003: 151). Clearly embryos and fetuses which are at home in women's wombs where they are 'hidden, secret' cross the canny/uncanny border when they are depicted ex utero. Much like 'revenants, spirits and ghosts,' they visit us from another world (Freud 1003: 148).[2]

Reactions to these dolls demonstrate that whether 'persons and things,… impressions, processes and situations' (Freud 2003: 135) are experienced as 'canny' or 'uncanny' depends on the eye of the beholder. Both terms refer to the stimulation or evocation of feelings, and people respond differently. While the makers and purchasers of memorial dolls find the life-likeness comforting, as evident from the testimonials on Dearborne's website; for others, even those who have suffered a pregnancy loss such as myself, they may instead arouse feelings of 'dread and creeping horror' (Freud 1949: 368).

2 As Mantel (2003, quoted in Peel and Cain, this volume) points out, in addition to children lost to miscarriage, some of those who are 'aborted or ... simply fail to materialize … [may] become ghosts within our lives.'

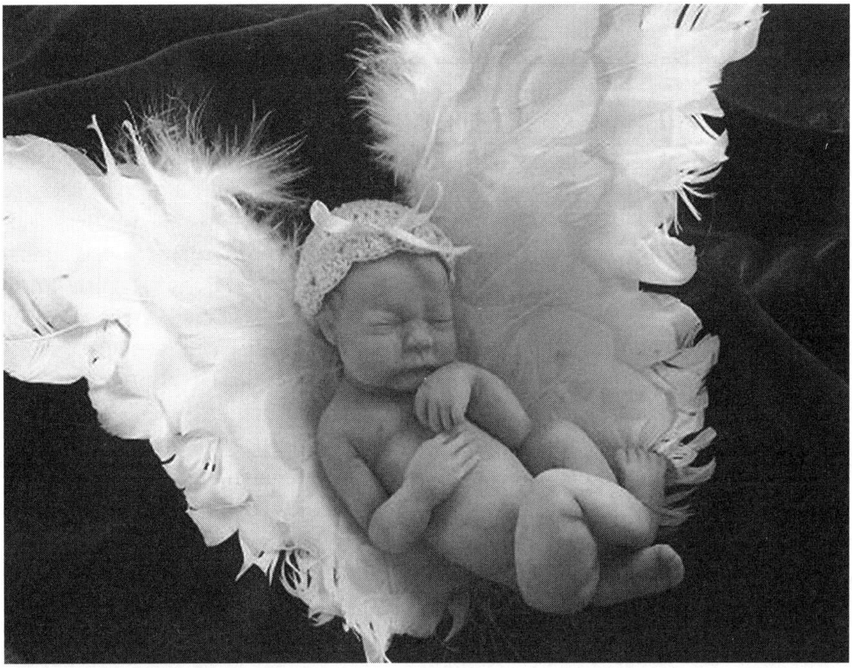

Figure 10.1 Sculpture by Jennifer Stocks

Source: http: //mytangiblepeace.webs.com/memorialartdolls.htm, permission by artist.

Conclusions

Despite how common pregnancy losses are, in the U.S. they are overwhelmingly experienced as abnormal (Layne 2004). Following a traumatic loss, members of pregnancy loss support groups find themselves in frightening, unchartered territory. Most of the frequently asked questions (FAQs) addressed on SHARE's website address parents' concerns about normality. Questions include, 'I feel like I am sad all the time. Is this *normal*? Is it *normal* to feel like I am going crazy? Is it *normal* to feel so tired?' Answers reassure parents that what they are feeling is normal. For example, the response to a question about resuming physical intimacy with one's partner is, 'Being hesitant *is normal*.' And as for returning to work, parents are advised, 'It is *normal* to have feelings of confusion, crying, having difficult days, or having trouble concentrating. Grief can make a *normal* day of work unbearable' (SHARE accessed May 27, 2011, emphases added). Despite these assurances that their feelings of grief are normal, and as much as bereaved parents may long for a return to the normal, they know it is unattainable. One bereaved mother explains her loss felt like being picked up by a tornado and dropped down 'in a totally different place … unable to find [her] way back to the place [she] had been before. That place no longer exists' (Daniels 1988). Furthermore, some fear it, as regaining normalcy would mean that they had gotten over, or forgotten, their dearly beloved baby.

In the face of their baby's absence, bereaved parents use poetic license to create a 'fable' of their child to share with others, including sometimes choosing the sex of miscarried 'babies' so that they may refer to them by name and thereby increase the 'plausibility' of their family story or by having photos retouched so as to make their experience appear more 'normal' and hence socially acceptable to others. But, in addition to altering the facts to make their experience jibe more with social norms, bereaved parents have attempted to broaden the definition of a 'normal family' to include miscarried or stillborn babies. Collectively, they have had some success as evidenced in the much greater availability of support resources for bereaved parents than there was when the first support groups were established in the mid-1970s (Layne 2006) as well as the federally-sanctioned Pregnancy Loss Awareness Day and Month, and 'Missing Angel Bills' in many states. But some of their efforts to attain social acceptance and legitimacy for their non-normative families backfire; some feel their practices are 'creepy' and 'bizarre' and evoke feelings of 'repulsion and distress' (Freud 2003: 123). Examples of this can be seen in reactions to the display pictures of miscarried or stillborn infants in workplaces where it is 'normal' for people to display photos of their 'normal' families.[3] One woman told me of a secretary who had framed sonogram images of each of her several miscarriages prominently displayed on her desk. The rest of the staff were 'horrified' by what seemed to them a 'bizarre' (and some felt, 'disgusting') behavior (Layne 2004). Similarly, a bereaved grandmother (Zorn 2001) reports that she kept finding the silver-framed photograph of her daughter holding her stillborn grandson face down on the credenza in her office (Layne 2003). The efforts of bereaved parents (and grandparents) to keep their dead babies present as a vital part of their family life are experienced by others as disturbing and out-of-place. Dead babies, they believe should be 'kept secret and hidden' and 'locked away within the house' (Freud 2003: 132, 133).

I conclude that members of the pregnancy loss support movement are forging new forms of families and that their efforts to do so can best be understood in the context of other emerging family including single mothers by choice, two-mom and two-dad families, surrogate mothers, and new figurations of older forms of family formations such as adoption. Bereaved parents, like single mothers by choice, and gay parents are exercising the creative freedoms available to Americans (at least those of certain means) to create new modes of kinship, including innovative kin terms, roles, rituals, and relationships. Empowered by new technologies and the 1960s rights movements, they feel entitled to make things up as they go along.

3 This reaction can also be inferred from some of the comments posted on the Facebook page, Remembering Our Babies, to the photographs of Dearborn's sculptures. One woman said she planned on ordering one and then will 'PROUDLY show it off.... If they don't like it, too bad, I have to see their baby pics all the time. They can see my Sculpture' (emphasis in original). (www.facebook.com/home.php#!/permalink.php?story_fbid=10150130011570741&id=56401190740).

They grant themselves poetic license, not just to make their family lives appear to conform to social norms, but to challenge those norms.

Acknowledgements

I am most indebted to my colleague and friend, Ellen Esrock, for recommending the cluster of concepts used in this chapter and actually providing curb-side delivery of Freud's essay and to G.J. Barker-Benfield for his many and varied intellectual and material contributions. This chapter is part of the comparative study which was presented at the ESRC-funded seminar 'Consumption and Contested Motherhood Identities' in Edinburgh in 2010, thanks to Stephanie O'Donohue.

References

Allen, M. and Marks, S. 1993. *Miscarriage: Women Sharing From the Heart*. New York: John Wiley & Sons.

Anonymous. 2010. Milestones. *Sharing*, 19(1), 5.

Campbell, H. 1992. The Picnic Basket. *UNITE Notes*, 11(1), 5.

Daniels, B.A. 1988. When My Baby Died, in *Bittersweet..hellogoodbye: A Resource in Planning Farewell Rituals When a Baby Dies*, edited by Sister J.M. Lamb. Belleville, Ill.: Charis Communications, 15.

Deloge, W. 2010. Milestones. *Sharing*, 19(1): 4.

Douglas, M. 1966. *Purity and Danger: An Analysis of the Concepts of Pollution and Taboo*. London: Routledge and Kegan Paul.

Fiorello, J. 2010. Birthdays. *Sharing*, 19(1): 5.

Franklin, S. 1997. *Embodied Progress: A Cultural Account of Assisted Conception*. London: Routledge.

Freud, S. 1949. The Uncanny, in *Sigmund Freud, Collected Papers, Volume IV*, translated by J. Riviere. London: The Hogarth Press, 368-407.

Freud, S. 2003. *The Uncanny*. Translated by D. Mclintock. New York: Penguin.

Freud, S. Nd. The Uncanny. [Online]. Available at: http: //www-rohan.sdsu.edu/~amtowcr/uncanny.html (accessed 1 December 2006).

Hirstein, W. 2006. *Brain Fiction: Self-Deception and the Riddle of Confabulation*. MIT Press.

Jones, J. 1992. Family Portraits. *UNITE Notes*, 11(2), 4.

Lammert, C. and Friedeck, S. (Compilers) 1997. *Angelic Presence: Short Stories of Solace and Hope after the Loss of a Baby*. Salt Lake: Richard Paul Evans Publishing Company.

Layne, L.L. 1996. 'Never Such Innocence Again': Irony, Nature and Technoscience in Narratives of Pregnancy Loss, in *Comparative Studies in Pregnancy Loss*, edited by R. Cecil. Oxford: Berg Publishers, 131-152.

Layne, L.L. 2000a. 'He was a Real Baby with Baby Things': A Material Culture Analysis of Personhood and Pregnancy Loss. *Journal of Material Culture*, 5(3), 321-345.

Layne, L.L. 2000b. Baby Things as Fetishes?: Memorial Goods, Simulacra, and the 'Realness' Problem of Pregnancy Loss, in *Ideologies and Technologies of Motherhood*, edited by H. Ragoné and F. Winddance Twine. NY: Routledge, 111-138.

Layne, L.L. 2001. 'I Remember the Day I Shopped for your Layette': Goods, Fetuses and Feminism in the Context of Pregnancy Loss, reprinted in *Consumption*, Critical Concepts in the Social Sciences Series, edited by D. Miller. London: Routledge, 286-318.

Layne, L.L. 2003. *Motherhood Lost: A Feminist Account of Pregnancy Loss in America*. New York: Routledge.

Layne, L.L. 2004. Making Memories: Trauma, Choice, and Consumer Culture in the Case of Pregnancy Loss, in *Consuming Motherhood* edited by J.S. Taylor, L.L. Layne and D.F. Wozniak. New Brunswick: Rutgers University Press, 122-138.

Layne, L.L. 2006a. Pregnancy and Infant Loss Support: A New, Feminist, American, Patient Movement? *Social Science & Medicine*, 62(3), 602-613.

Layne, L.L. 2006b. 'Your Child Deserves a Name': Possessive Individualism and the Politics of Memory in Pregnancy Loss, in *Tropes of Entanglement: Towards an anthropology of names and naming*, edited by G. vom Bruck and B. Bodenhorn. Cambridge: Cambridge University Press, 31-50.

Layne, LL. (forthcoming) The use of consumer goods and services to manage the contested motherhood identities in the context of pregnancy loss and intentionally father-absent families, in *Motherhood, Markets, and Consumption: The Making of Mothers in Contemporary Western Culture*, edited by O'Donohoe, M. Hogg, P. Maclaran, L. Martens, and L. Stevens (eds.) Routledge.

Lewin, E. 1993. *Lesbian Mothers: Accounts of Gender in American Culture*. Ithaca: Cornell University Press.

Lustig, D.F. 2004. Baby Pictures: Family, Consumerism and Exchange among Teen Mothers in the USA. *Childhood*, 11(2): 175-193.

Mamo, L. 2007. *Queering Reproduction: Achieving Pregnancy in the Age of Technoscience*. Durham: Duke University Press.

Ohlson, K. 2010. Just a Memory Before You Sleep Forever. [Online]. Available at: http: //www.miller-mccune.com/culture/just-a-memory-before-you-sleep-forever-17742/ [accessed 1 February 2012].

Ragoné, H. 1994. *Surrogate Motherhood: Conception in the Heart*. Boulder: Westview Press.

Schneider, J. (Alexander's Grammy) 1996. Grammy's Grief. *SHARE Newsletter*, 5(2), 6-8.

Seven Days. 2007. *Slide Show: Memorial Dolls*. [Online, 8 August]. Available at: http: //7dvt.com/aux/multimedia/slideshows/080807-memorialdolls/. Cathy Resmer, Producer [accessed 1 February 2012].

Smith, S. 1999. My Story and the Importance of Rituals. *SHARING*, 8(4), 8.

Thompson, C. 2005. *Making Parents: The Ontological Choreography of Reproductive Technologies*. Cambridge: MIT Press.

Thompson, L. 2007. A Vermont Artist Finds Healing, and an Income, with Lifelike Infant Sculptures. *Seven Days*, Aug 8.

Threads of Remembrance. [Online]. Available at: www.meriter.com/content/?cm_id=357 (accessed 7 June 2011).

Young, D. 2009. Alina's Signs of Love. *Sharing*, 18(5), 10.

Chapter 11

Baby Gardens: A Privilege or Predicament?

Kate Woodthorpe

While the study of memorialization – why people do it, where and how – has taken off in recent years, very little is known about the practice of memorializing nearly viable foetuses (NVFs), babies, infants and young children (see Layne and Davidsson Bremborg, this volume). In the UK this is despite a substantial growth in the support available for bereaved parents and siblings through networks and charities such as Sands and the Childhood Bereavement Network, as well as research on the experience of being bereaved of a child (for example, Riches and Dawson 2000).

Elsewhere, in relation to the services provided by UK cemeteries and crematoria, through their Charter for the Bereaved (ICCM 2009) and guidance on the sensitive disposal of foetal remains (ICCM 2011), the Institute of Cemetery and Crematorium Management (ICCM) has advocated that bereaved parents should be allowed a choice in how the remains of their child should be managed and their existence memorialized. The aforementioned Charter also endorses the principle that there should be a distinct area for parents to visit within a cemetery.

This chapter considers the provision of baby gardens from the perspective of those who are tasked with providing and managing these spaces. Specifically, it examines what actually takes place in these spaces and how the activity is interpreted by cemetery staff. First, it suggests that through the separation of a distinct space for babies and children, participants see baby gardens as creating a bounded community for lost offspring. Rather than the metaphor of 'sleep' being adopted in this space to refer to those interred there, as seen in previous research I have conducted in relation to buried adults (Woodthorpe 2010a), the metaphor of a 'nursery' may be more appropriate here Protection and companionship feature in this metaphor. Following on from these theoretical explanations, the chapter suggests that those tasked with managing baby gardens are actually managing expectations in a climate of 'rights', which are complicated by the ongoing, continuing, bonds that parents can have with the children interred in the site. Overall, the chapter shows how baby gardens reveal a changing attitude towards the treatment of, and grieving for, nearly viable foetuses (NVFs), babies, infants and young children, which in itself is indicative of wider shifting approaches to the expression of grief in public.

An Overview of Memorialization

In recent years the academic study of memorialization has gathered apace. Within the amorphous field of death studies, it has been associated with meaning-making (Simone 2010), the art of writing (Goodhead 2010) and the strength of personal relationships and social values (Gibson 2008). Memorializing activity after high profile deaths, such as that of Diana, Princess of Wales in 1997 has also garnered significant interest, particularly for sociologists in relation to the public expression of grief (see Walter 2008). In some cases the starting point for analysing memorializing practices is the position that they are 'excessive' (Doss 2010: 13). Elsewhere, the term 'spontaneous shrines' has been coined by folklorist Santino (2006) to describe the creation of unplanned areas of commemorative activity.

One reason for this increase in attention is the inter-disciplinary nature of studying the activity itself. Certainly, memorializing dead people has captured the imagination of those scholars with an interest in material culture (Hockey et al. 2010), human geography (Maddrell and Sidaway 2010), and history (Bleyen 2010), to name a few.

Despite this burgeoning interest, very little is known about the practice of memorializing NVFs, babies, infants and young children. While there have been a number of insightful and detailed accounts from scholars regarding the changing attitude(s) towards the death of babies, children and young people in their respective native countries of Belgium (Bleyen 2010) Denmark (Sørenson 2011) and the Netherlands (Peelen 2009: 2011), there is a particular dearth of insight into UK memorializing activity for NVFs, pre-term, stillbirth, infant and young children. This chapter intends to address this gap in the literature, drawing on research conducted with staff tasked with managing the spaces in which interment and memorialization takes place in the UK.

Research Methods

The research underpinning this chapter is a series of interviews with those who have been associated with cemeteries and crematoria. Building on my previous research on how memorialization is managed within a cemetery (Woodthorpe 2008, 2010a), I conducted 10 interviews with cemetery and crematoria managers. All were asked about their experiences and observations of the provision of facilities for bereaved parents.

The decision to focus on those who work in cemeteries was principally guided by pragmatism and access. From my own experience of conducting research in cemeteries, approaching recently bereaved people can be difficult (see Woodthorpe 2011) and thus discussing experiences with parents bereaved of a baby was – for a project of this size – potentially too complex and emotionally demanding for one person. For this reason, the scope of the research does not include examining *why* parents may be memorializing their deceased offspring in their own words.

Rather, it examines the perspective of those tasked with creating and managing these areas in order to generate a basic understanding of the issues – outlined in this chapter – with a view to possibly extending the research in the future to explore the experience of parents themselves.

To note, in terms of research ethics all participants were provided with an information sheet and asked for their written consent. In keeping with the British Sociological Association Ethical Statement of Practice (2002), letters are used to identify participants and protect their identity.

Memorializing Babies

As already outlined, little is documented about how the remains of NVFs, babies, infants and children in the UK have been managed and how their lives have been commemorated in cemeteries. Historically, stillborn babies and infants were typically buried with adults, mainly placed in the coffin of an unrelated woman. However, since the 1990s there has been a change in attitude towards the way in which the remains of stillborn babies and babies are handled. Most local authorities now provide a designated area in a cemetery or crematoria within their catchment area specifically for NVFs, babies and/or children. Many also provide funeral services for stillborn babies and/or babies.

There are several potential drivers for the change in approach from local authorities. During the early years of establishing baby gardens in the 1990s, there was a move towards greater collaboration between NHS Trusts and local authorities in determining the services available to newly bereaved parents. Several years later, the introduction of the Human Tissue Authority Code of Practice (2009) established standards for disposing of foetal remains (see Code 5). Around the same time the aforementioned ICCM Charter for the Bereaved (2009) established good practice standards for the provision of baby gardens. These standards were underpinned by guidance set out in the ICCM's guidance on the disposal of fetal remains (2011) and Royal College of Nursing guidance for nurses and midwives on the disposal of foetal remains (2007). All three documents made reference to disposal choice for the parents, treating the deceased offspring as an individual death, and offering appropriately 'respectful' services. Finally, and perhaps most significantly, were the campaigns and efforts by charities such as Sands and bereaved parents themselves, particularly bereaved mothers, who have been increasingly vocal about their experiences of loss, alongside work on the quality of care provided by midwives (Mander 2005) and academic work on the politics of reproduction (such as Layne 2003). As one participant told me in their interview:

> [providing a section for babies is] not something we've always done, but I think it started because there was a need for it. Mothers were coming to us and saying 'I don't want my baby in there, I want my baby to have its own grave'. (B)

This emphasis on, and demand for, individual burial echoes a shifting late-modern emphasis on privileging individual's experiences of loss and grief (Walter 1994, 1999) and has led to the establishment of procedures for treating, handling and managing NVFs and stillborn children (as well as babies) as individuals. As a result, parents are now typically given the option to deal with the remains of their lost offspring as an individual, including the choice of cremation or interment (see Royal College of Nursing 2007). One outcome of this change in approach has been the exponential growth in the provision of baby gardens within cemeteries across the UK. As advocated in the Charter for the Bereaved (ICCM 2009), the majority of cemeteries and many crematoria now have a designated interment area for babies and young children. These areas are usually bounded in some way by trees, hedges or low walls, and often contain a focal point such as a bench, statue or memorial. They often also have a slightly varied policy on memorialization and maintenance compared to the rest of the cemetery, with a 'lighter touch' in the removal of artefacts left by visitors. A result of this lighter touch is the extent to which the baby garden can become full of artefacts, which on first sight can appear similar to a children's nursery.

Creating a Nursery

The creation of memorial sites or 'shrines' following an unexpected death, often at the roadside as the result of a road traffic accident, have become commonplace in contemporary Western societies. Shrines are not confined to highways however, and can be found in many cemeteries throughout the UK. One reason for this was given by a participant who believed that the near-universal adoption of the lawn grave[1] (see Rugg (2006) for a history) has led to the need for bereaved people to personalize the grave through the leaving of mementoes:

> We find it with all graves, the modern lawn memorial looks like everybody else's and it's taken off a shelf, stuck on the computer and the letters are cut. So what do people do? (A)

Within baby gardens it is typical that either a small low laying grave marker or plaque will be provided to identify the child. The options for markers are usually dependent on the way in which remains are interred; be they buried in individual plots or in communal graves. What does happen more often than not, however, is the proliferation of more transient and temporary artefacts in the baby garden, as the parents visit and leave mementoes (the reasons for which are considered in Peelen (2011) and later in this chapter). In reference to their own UK site, one participant noted:

---

1 The lawn grave memorial is typically a simple rectangular headstone (with or without kerbset) placed in a long straight line of plots.

> We got to a point where we had an entire area covered in floral tributes and toys and windmills and teddy bears and if you allow these things to develop they become shrines. (I)

Another told me:

> I know all too well, all my years working in cemeteries, how that parents, when they've lost a baby, it's obviously a devastating thing, and that the grave, the plot, becomes a shrine. And they want to adorn that grave with things that people wouldn't normally put on graves. So you will get a profusion of balloons, teddy bears and toys, windmills, glittery things and lanterns. You name it. (F)

A consequence of this memorializing activity is that often the baby garden appears to the visitor as a colourful, ornate and youthful area; it is a highly visible community of babies, which participants felt that parents got a lot of comfort from. While previous research (Woodthorpe 2010b) has shown that the tendency to refer to the deceased person as residing in a grave as 'sleeping' or 'lying down' is not uncommon, in the context of baby sections the metaphor used by participants was not one of a bedroom. Rather, the interred babies were referred to as being part of a community – together – as if in in a crèche or nursery. As one participant (J) noted, 'it is comforting to know that babies are buried together.' Participant E reflected on why this may be the case:

> Children are different to adults and children need to be separated from adults, in death as in life … Because after all children don't like being on their own, they're tribal by nature sort of thing, part of the growing up process. (E)

Another participant commented similarly:

> A lone headstone is more distressing than having your child in amongst others, you know, they're alone. (D)

In talking about the reasons behind having a separate section for babies, one participant noted that their own local authority's decision had been influenced by a perceived desire for babies and children to be together:

> I think the rationale behind the burial sections [here] was to provide an area exclusively for the burial of babies/children under 14. It was probably believed that families would prefer an area where babies and children could be together, although they could choose to have a grave in any part of the cemetery if they preferred. (G)

The concept of community and companionship in baby gardens permeated all interviews in one form or another, specifically in the way in which the baby garden could be, and *should* be, separated from the other areas of the cemetery containing adult burials. For example, participant E commented that they felt that a baby garden should be contained, bounded by walls:

> It [the baby garden] should have boundaries. Whether that is a low wall with a gate, whether you plant a hedge, or whether it's obvious because you tarmac paths and grass, *but it is important to separate it.* (E) [*emphasis* added]

One participant reflected on the boundaries that surround the areas in which babies and children reside when alive, and how this carries over into death:

> I think there's something about, children have playgrounds, they have schools that are boundaried aren't they? It [the baby garden] had no boundary, and I think there's something about [it now it has a boundary], their families know that this is their area. This is the children's area. (D)

So why may boundaries be so important in this context? Principally, boundaries are a way of symbolically and practically outlining the location of deceased people and protecting the living from the dead, as was the original intention of the modern urban cemetery. Data for this project indicated however that rather than protecting the living from the dead, bounded baby gardens had a function in protecting the deceased babies from the world around them. Perceived as vulnerable and defenceless residents, one participant noted that when examining the creation of a new baby area, families had welcomed the idea of the new area being situated next to the war memorial section:

> I didn't think they'd like being near the soldiers. But actually they said they really did like that because it was like they were protecting them. And they had the formality of the soldiers, because it's the Commonwealth War Graves Commission, they look after it. So that was very formal, and then you have the baby's next to it, which was a big contrast. (H)

Furthermore, by putting babies *together* one participant commented that they had seen a decline in requests for bereaved parents to be buried with their deceased child:

> There is evidence that some parents get a lot of benefit from knowing that their baby lies with others, in one place … there will be those that purchase a full size grave for baby to be buried so that mum and dad can be buried there in future years. You tend to find that when a baby garden is introduced that that decreases. (A)

According to this participant, by being located with other babies meant parents no longer felt the desire to be buried with their child as their offspring was already being protected and accompanied by the other babies surrounding them.

Ascribing Value

One significant aspect of this idea of protection is the way in which the baby garden demarcates a special status to the child, as *belonging* to a clearly defined community. This status is not just associated with the space in which the baby resides however; it reflects the way in which their non-normative death is being increasingly recognized within UK society. The physical union of these babies in their distinct space serves to sequestrate – that is distinguish – their non-normative death (as opposed to an older adult who died at the end of a relatively long life), and by association it delineates their parents as people bereaved of an exceptional death. This is a deliberate response to the 'devalued' status that has typically accompanied death at the beginning of life (Layne 2003, Lovell 1997), and is a highly visible contribution to the growing social recognition of the impact of loss at this stage of life.

There are implications for this growing recognition of loss however. One consequence of being accorded this special status for parents, from the perspective of the staff I interviewed, is the accompaniment of an exceptional 'right' to commemorate their deceased offspring as they wish.

Managing Expectations: The Language of 'Rights'

A key aspect of the cemetery manager's job in maintaining a section for babies was identified by all as getting the balance between allowing personal expression through artefacts while ensuring the site was safe to enter and relatively straightforward to maintain. Several participants spoke from experience of not managing expectations sufficiently, and then finding they were unable to adequately look after their site. For example, in describing the problems of pruning the boundary hedges around the baby section one participant noted,

> If there's a teddybear in the hedge, you don't know who it belongs to. And it's not really doing any harm, until it's time to cut the hedge. And it might be by then that that teddybear has gone. But it might be that it's turned into 10 teddybears. So, it's horrible [when you have to remove them]. (D)

One way of negotiating the potential proliferation of memorializing activity that is afforded by the non-normative deaths that the babies represent is a clear set of guidelines over how the area will be managed. As one participant noted,

> I think if you're starting a baby area you start it and make it very clear that you will follow a certain process, and give people a clear understanding of what to expect. (I)

Other participants endorsed this view, stating that the provision of clear guidelines and their consistent implementation was key in ensuring that a baby garden was not hazardous for visitors, nor too unwieldy to maintain.

As to causes for the proliferation of the idea of having a 'right' to memorialize, one participant linked memorializing activity within baby gardens to a broader social shift in expectations about what someone has a 'right' to do when bereaved:

> People's attitudes have changed. When I first came in to the cemetery service 30 years ago, the cemetery superintendent who you worked for was on a par with the local bank manager. And if he said out, people went. They didn't argue with him. Now it's different. People challenge. People know their rights don't they? I'm not saying that's wrong, just people's attitudes have changed. (A)

The idea that in the twenty first century the experience of bereavement is a relatively rare life experience (and a bereavement of a child even more so) has meant that there has been a change in attitude towards the expression of grief in public (see Walter 2008). Out of this has evolved a change in approach to memorializing deceased people more generally, whereby individuals can memorialize as they wish. One participant referred to this growing trend as people creating 'D-I-Y memorials':

> It's that notion that people feel that if they've lost someone they have that right to, not claim the place where they actually died, but to claim where their remains have been placed. With that right they want to adorn it how they wish. And I think people like to adorn lawn graves now very much how they like to adorn their front gardens and their homes. There is all this paraphernalia, all these deals down at B&Q for these little fences and little lanterns, you name it! And that's what people use. It's their D-I-Y memorial. (F)

This sentiment was echoed by another participant who commented,

> 100 years ago people used to see rules and regulations and abide by them. But now they see the other things that are out there, and as they put it quite often to me, 'it's my way of grieving, I want to do things to remember my loved one' (C)

For babies, a life that was not lived, these D-I-Y memorials – as an expression of a right to express 'grief how I want' – become both a source of tension for those tasked with managing the space in which they are located, and a method of communication for the parents. In this way, participants in this research hypothesized, leaving artefacts for deceased babies and children is regarded by many parents as a way of continuing the parent/child bond.

Continuing Bonds

So what of the interpretation of participants as to the potential reasons for the practice of visiting and leaving mementoes in the baby section? Several participants indicated that there are potent reasons for leaving artefacts, not least as a form of 'gift giving':

> We have it where they [parents] bring pocket money. They put pocket money down. And Christmas dinners, and birthday cakes. They're left there for some time and then we take them off. (F)

> Most people do want to cover that space [the plot] with bits and bobs, tend the grave and leave things. People tend to want to leave balloons for birthdays. And other children like to come and play with the bits. (H)

The idea of giving presents to deceased people, particularly at the site of their remains, has long been present in anthropological insights into the relationship between those alive and those who have died (see Bloch and Parry 1982). As noted in the opening sections of this chapter, sociological and psychological theory have recently begun to contribute to this discussion. Indeed, my own work has drawn on psychological concepts of bereavement and continuing bonds to examine the reasoning behind memorializing activity (Woodthorpe 2010a). Verifying the occurrence of (lay) psychologizing within the cemetery, the idea that presents are given to the deceased baby at the site of their grave was articulated by one participant as a form of continuing the parental bond with the baby:

> It's all about continuing bonds isn't it? … By putting something back on that gravestone that you know was important for that person in there, it's a tribute of love isn't it? And it's like giving a present. There's as much in giving as there is in receiving. And the grieving person feels like they're giving something, it's their way of talking to the deceased. It's their partner, their child or whatever. It's that unseen tie. And quite often it will be things that were in the house … I'll take this as they would have liked to have that with them. (D)

As a way of visibly demonstrating the tie between parent and child, the memorialization of NVFs, babies, infants and young children contributes to the valuing of their non-normative death. This leaves those tasked with managing these spaces in a tenuous position however, as on the one hand they are facilitating the visible material expression of grief for parents who have lost a child through providing a space for interment and commemoration. On the other hand, this space needs to be policed to ensure that it is safe to enter and relatively straightforward to maintain. In other words, they are tasked with 'containing' the memorialization of babies.

Conclusion: Containing Memorialization

This chapter has hinted throughout at tensions as to the control of memorialization. In a public and shared space such as a baby garden, unlimited memorialization cannot be allowed lest the site become unwieldy to maintain and hazardous for visitors. The issue for the participants in this research thus relates to their role in setting expectations with regard to memorialization and the consistent management of the space in which parents are permitted to commemorate their deceased offspring. This presents an inherent tension between their desire to recognize the parents' loss and their associated 'right' to grieve, alongside the need to restrain that material expression of grief. As noted earlier in this chapter, one way to manage this tension is to provide clear and consistent guidelines on what is permitted within the baby garden. The extent to which these guidelines are successful needs to be examined in future research and, certainly, more could be learnt from research with the parents and families who receive these guidelines. Furthermore, the personal sense of unease that many of the participants indicated when talking about removing artefacts from baby gardens suggests that this is far from a straightforward process for those tasked with the job.

This chapter has detailed some of the issues faced by those charged with providing and managing baby sections in cemeteries. Regarded as good practice, the creation of distinct baby sections can be seen metaphorically as an attempt to create a bounded nursery that provides the babies with company and protects them from the wider world. One result of creating separate sections however can be a proliferation of mementoes on graves, accompanied by an expectation that the gift-giver is permitted to do so as a 'right' associated with their bereavement. Through talking with individuals who have had much experience of these spaces, this chapter needs to be regarded as an opening gambit in terms of examining and theorizing the practice of memorializing babies. There is a dearth of academic insight into these practices in the UK, and much still to be learnt from the parents themselves about why they do it, their relationship to the deceased baby, and the space in which the baby resides.

References

Bleyen, J. 2010. The materialities of absence after stillbirth: historical perspectives, in *The Matter of Death: space, place and materiality*, edited by J. Hockey, C.Komaromy and K. Woodthorpe. Basingstoke: Palgrave Macmillan, 69-84.

Bloch, M. and Parry, J. (eds) 1982. *Death and the Regeneration of Life*. Cambridge: Cambridge University Press.

British Sociological Association. 2002. *Statement of Ethical Practice for the British Sociological Association (March 2002)* [Online] Available at: http://www.britsoc.co.uk/equality/Statement+Ethical+Practice.htm [accessed: 25 November 2011].

Doss, E. 2010. *Memorial Mania: Public feeling in America*. London: University of Chicago.

Gibson, M. 2008. *Objects of the Dead*. Melbourne: Melbourne University Press.

Goodhead, A. 2010. A textual analysis of memorials written by bereaved individuals and families in a hospital context. *Mortality*, 15(4), 323-339.

Hockey, J., Komaromy, C. and Woodthorpe, K. 2010. *The Matter of Death: Space, Place and Materiality*. Basingstoke: Palgrave Macmillan.

Human Tissue Authority 2009. *Code of Practice 5: Disposal of human tissue*. [Online] Available at: http://www.hta.gov.uk/legislationpoliciesandcodesofpractice/codesofpractice/code5disposal.cfm?FaArea1=customwidgets.content_view_1&cit_id=724&cit_parent_cit_id=713 [accessed: 25 November 2011].

Institute of Cemetery and Crematorium Management (ICCM) 2009. *Charter for the Bereaved*. [Online] Available at: http:/www.iccm-uk.com/iccm/library/Reference%20Charter.doc [accessed: 25 November 2011].

Institute of Cemetery and Crematorium Management (ICCM) 2011. *The Sensitive Disposal of Fetal Remains: policy and guidance for burial and cremation authorities and companies*. [Online] Available at: http://www.iccm-uk.com/iccm/library/FetalRemainsPolicyAug2011FINAL.pdf [accessed: 25 November 2011].

Layne, L.L. 2003. *Motherhood Lost: a feminist account of pregnancy loss in America*. New York: Routledge.

Lovell, A. 1997. Death at the beginning of life, in *Death, Gender and Ethnicity*, edited by D. Field, J. Hockey and N. Small. London: Routledge, 29-51.

Maddrell, A. and Sidaway, J. (eds). 2010. *Deathscapes*. Farnham, Surrey: Ashgate.

Mander, R. 2005. *Loss and Bereavement in Childbearing*. London: Taylor and Francis.

Peelen, J. 2009. Reversing the Past: monuments for stillborn children. *Mortality*, 14(2), 173-186.

Peelen, J. 2011. *Between Birth and Death: rituals of pregnancy loss in the Netherlands*. Unpublished PhD thesis. Nijmegen: Radboud Universiteit.

Riches, G. and Dawson, P. 2000. *An Intimate Loneliness: supporting bereaved parents and siblings*. Buckingham: Open University Press.

Royal College of Nursing. 2007. *Sensitive Disposal of all Fetal Remains: guidance for nurses and midwives*. London: Royal College of Nursing.

Rugg, J. 2006. Lawn cemeteries: the emergence of a new landscape of death. *Urban History*, 33, 213-233.

Santino, J. 2006. *Spontaneous Shrines and the Public Memorialization of Death*. Basingstoke: Palgrave Macmillan.

Simone, C. 2010. Memorializing the suicide victim: 'walking the walk', in *The Matter of Death: space, place and materiality*, edited by J. Hockey, C. Komaromy and K. Woodthorpe. Basingstoke: Palgrave Macmillan, 178-194.

Sørenson, T.F. 2011. Sweet dreams: biographical blanks and the commemoration of children. *Mortality*, 16(2), 161-175.

Walter, T. 1994. *The Revival of Death*. London: Routledge.

Walter, T. 1999. *On Bereavement: the culture of grief.* Maidenhead: Open University Press.

Walter, T. 2008. The new public mourning, in *Handbook of Bereavement Research and Practice: advances in theory and intervention*, edited by M.S. Stroebe, R.O. Hansson, H. Schut, and W. Stroebe. Washington, DC: American Psychological Association, 241-262.

Woodthorpe, K. 2008. *Negotiating ambiguity and uncertainty in the contemporary cemetery*. Unpublished PhD thesis. Sheffield: University of Sheffield.

Woodthorpe, K. 2010a. Private grief in public spaces: Interpreting memorialization in the contemporary cemetery, in *The Matter of Death: space, place and materiality*, edited by J. Hockey, C. Komaromy, and K. Woodthorpe. Basingstoke: Palgrave Macmillan, 117-132.

Woodthorpe, K. 2010b. Revisiting taboo: Buried bodies in an East London Cemetery, in *Deathscapes*, edited by A. Maddrell and J. Sidaway. Farnham, Surrey: Ashgate, 57-74.

Woodthorpe, K. 2011. Researching death: methodological reflections on the management of critical distance. *International Journal of Social Research Methodology*, 14(2), 99-109.

Chapter 12
The Memorialization of Stillbirth in the Internet Age

Anna Davidsson Bremborg

On a Swedish Internet community site for parents, I found a message posted by a mother asking for party tips for her daughter. It was the type of question that is very common on these kinds of sites. However, this time, it was for the memorial party on the first anniversary of her stillborn daughter:

> When you have a children's party usually the kids get a candy bag when leaving. Most people coming are adults, so I thought I would give them a (memorial) candy bag. Some candy, a poem, a candle perhaps. Does anybody have any other tips?[1]

The mother got several suggestions: balloons with the daughter's name on, a photograph of the daughter, and bubbles. Another idea was to write the name on a piece of paper and stick it to a candle. This reminded another mother (who wrote a reply) about her daughter's funeral, where guests could write messages on pieces of paper and put them into a pot by the coffin. When the coffin had been lowered, all messages were thrown into the grave. Maybe she could do something similar now?

I will take this story as the starting point for a discussion about how grief after stillbirth is talked about today. In this chapter, I want to bring together three components that are present in the excerpt above: discourses of grief after stillbirth, memorialization, and the Internet. With respect to the discourses of grief, I mean the text or talk about how you should or could grieve; in other words, the norms and values that are part of grieving following stillbirth. Memorialization refers, in this case, to the use of private rituals that follow a stillbirth. The Internet I regard as a virtual arena for communication and I primarily use open data sources including Web pages and discussion groups in my analysis here. The Chapter discusses the value changes regarding grief and memorialization that can be observed on the Internet following a stillbirth.

---

1 Author's translation from Swedish. The URL has been protected for ethical reasons and is kept by the author.

Discourses of Grief

The legal terms of a stillbirth varies nationally and over time. In Sweden, there was a legal change in 2008 (SFS 2008: 207), when the term stillborn was changed in the national civil registration law from 'dead after the end of the 28th pregnancy week' to 'dead after the end of the 22nd pregnancy week' (SFS 1991: 481). A stillborn, according to this definition, should be registered the same way as living babies. The change was in accordance with international practice, especially the recommendations from the World Health Organization in their statistical classification ICD-10 (WHO 1992). However, this change was also due to medical progress in the care of neonates where the survival is now nearly 80 per cent for children born between the end of the 22nd and 28th pregnancy week (Lagrådsremiss 2008). The legal change has consequences not only on mortality statistics but also on who is officially regarded to be a human being.

It is only during the last twenty to thirty years that grief after stillbirth has been acknowledged by hospital staff and caregivers. Many women who experienced a stillbirth during the larger part of the 20th century had their children taken away immediately after birth and got the advice to forget what had happen and try to get pregnant again (see both Bleyen and Komaromy, this volume). However, during the 1980s and early 1990s, practices within the hospital wards changed (Andersson Wretmark 1993, Rådestad et al. 1996). Parents are now advised to see, touch, and hold the child, as attachment to the child is regarded as being important for the grieving process (Rådestad 1999, Lundqvist 2003, Säflund 2003). The new practices have changed a lot for bereaved parents. It has become customary to have photographs taken of the stillborn baby, hand and footprints, and not least, embodied memories of the child such as having felt their weight and touched their faces, hands, and bodies (Rådestad et al. 1996, Riches & Dawson 1998, Godel 2007). Still, many parents experience a silence after stillbirth. The acknowledgement of the stillborn baby from the hospital staff in the immediate aftermath do not always have any parallels with reactions from relatives, friends, neighbours, work colleagues, and public authorities. After a few months, the parents are expected to be 'back on track' in their everyday lives.

Though acknowledgement of the child has changed within hospital care, it is primarily seen as the first important step in the grief process, with the aim of separating the parents and the child from each other. During the last ten years, this view of the grief process as a 'letting-go' of the dead has been questioned. Studies have shown that bereaved individuals have ongoing relations with dead people (Walter 1996, Hallam et al. 1999, Klass 1999, Grout and Romanoff 2000). Yet, these relations are not commonly discussed, as they are not always recognized as expressions of 'healthy grief'.

Memorialization

Grief is closely connected with religious rituals. In all cultures, in all times, death has been coped with through rituals and funerals have been the foremost studied ritual in anthropology (Davies 1997).

However, in northern Europe, official religion has been in decline for decades. Thus, it is relevant to ask whether the relationship between grief and ritual remains the same. Although many studies show that Europeans have a faith, this faith appears to be more private and personal (Davie 1994). In Sweden, a majority identify themselves as 'Christian in their own personal way' (Hamberg 2003, Bäckström et al. 2004) but this 'personal way' is difficult to measure statistically since it is, by nature, disparate. So while participation in official, traditional rituals such as church services is low, we know very little about the privately performed rituals that may be part of a personal faith and set of beliefs.

Heelas and Woodhead (2005) have declared that a spiritual revolution has taken place in late modern Western Societies, with a fundamental shift in the view of life. They see religion and spirituality as disparate concepts, defined by the teachings and life expectations. 'Religion' belongs to traditional churches, where lives are supposed to be lived in relation to a 'higher good' (God) and in accordance with stipulated duties. Life is lived through different roles, set by others. It is a 'life-as' religion. In the holistic milieus, which are growing, spirituality is distinct from this. It is a 'subjective-life forms of the sacred'. Spirituality is created by each individual and found within oneself. No one else decides what or how one should believe, and the authority is the inner self. So, religiosity has not necessarily disappeared, but the forms have changed, or as Heelas and Woodhead (2005) put it in the title of their book: 'religion is giving way to spirituality.'

If a spiritual revolution – or change – is taking place, we can assume great effects also for memorialization. Funeral rituals have become more individualized and personalized, something noted by all researchers today, and consequently, we must look more into the private sphere. The funeral is but one of many kinds of rituals taking place when someone has died. Rituals are performed in the home and by the grave site. This is not new but has been in much lesser degree observed.

However, to talk about rituals in the private sphere might be doubtful because it might lead the thoughts to structured rituals, with some kind of regulation or order. A more useful concept is ritualization, which Hallam and Hockey (2001, 179) point out 'is not confined to clearly demarcated phases of ritual but can be seen as a feature of "everyday" life, in which even the most mundane objects, such as clothing, can facilitate the work of memory.' Ritualization refers to, 'embodied acts that create links from different time and spaces' (2001: 181).

Within the wider concept of ritualization, it might be easier to catch new forms of religiosity without defining them as belonging to neither religion nor spirituality.

The Internet

We are living in a network society, Castells (2001) argues, and it is hard to prove the contrary. Even if Internet usage differs globally the World Wide Web has become a part of everyday life for many, not least for the parental age group. In Sweden, more than 80 per cent in the age group 25-44 years use a computer at least once per work day, and less than 5 per cent use it more seldom than once a month (SCB 2009). It is a place to find a recipe for dinner, watch a missed television program, book a ticket, and talk with a friend on the other side of the world, to mention just a few of the things that I have done myself in the last twenty-four hours.

From a sociological perspective, the Web is interesting with regards to the boundaries between private and public expressions of grief. The distinction usually made between the private sphere (the home and family) and the public sphere (work places, market places, and media, for example) seem to disappear, or at least to be blurred, on the Internet. Family home pages and blogs function as public diaries and photo albums, things that used to be very private. However, it is too easy to draw the conclusion that nothing is private anymore, and that 'that is a shame.' Such a view stems from the norm that things in the private sphere should be kept there. The reality is more complex. The private and personal on home pages and blogs is of major importance for showing authenticity, which is a virtue in the public sphere (Giddens 1991). At the same time, it is a construction of reality and of identity; what is written and published is a selection of life and identity, being conscious or unconscious. The private face on the Internet is a constructed and created identity. On the other hand, this could also be said about face-to-face-relations (Goffman 1968) and the difference might not be as large as one might think.

Results from a Study

By bringing together the three components: discourses of grief, memorialization, and the Internet, I will now point at some value changes in contemporary society. The Web will be used as the source of the study. Yet, this is not primarily a study of the Internet, but of how changes on the Internet point toward changes in social life more generally. I will use discussions and comments on home pages as mirrors of what could be said or portrayed in the public sphere. It is a discourse in which values and norms are revealed, questioned, and negotiated. Four aspects of grief will be discussed: a new parental identity, facilitated communication, photographs of the stillborn, and memorialization. They have all gotten legitimacy on the Internet and are in different aspects 'new' or point toward changed norms and values.

Angel Babies and Angel Parents

One significant aspect of being a parent of a dead child is the semantic identity problem: what is a bereaved parent? Davies (1997) points out this semantic problem for the English language and compares it with the Hebrew existence of words for bereaved parents, which are not only psychologically beneficial, but also carry strong political significance in a country where many parents have lost children serving in the Israeli army.

In previous years, new concepts have emerged for the stillborn, angel babies, and for their grieving parents, parents of angels or angel parents (also see Layne, this volume). These concepts have not reached official status, as they have not been accepted in the official Swedish Word List from 2006 (SAOL 2006) and a search at www.onelook.com, looking through 65 English dictionaries, did not give any references. However, the expressions are commonly used on the Internet and thus probably in the spoken language. One good indicator is the virtual community Facebook, where (on 1 July 2009) there were several groups with the name Angel Babies referring to stillborn children, some with more than a thousand members. Surprisingly though, it was, at the same time, not possible to find the words on the English version of Wiktionary, the online dictionary where everyone can add new words. The Swedish Wiktionary, though, had the word for angel parent (änglaförälder).

The use of the words angel babies and angel parents seems to be widespread enough to have legitimacy, even if the connotations are not clear-cut. An analysis of the usage of the Swedish words shows that these words are mainly used for stillborn babies and their parents, although, at times, children who have lived (for some weeks or years) and then died are included.

Obviously, the Internet precedes official language, as spoken language always does, but the occurrence also shows the need for these words, otherwise they would not have become so common. One reason is probably that the new words have larger implications than just the semantics. They identify a social situation and the agencies involved. The words distinguish the specific situation of grieving a stillborn, and they identify the parents as parents and the stillborn as a child. It not only makes talking about the situation easier but also highlights the grief of losing a child by giving it a name. It is a way of taking parents' grief seriously.

Having specific concepts for a life situation is also important for identity. In late modern society, identity construction is part of life. The answer to the question Who am I? is ongoing work, and words defining one's identity are essential.

Even if the word angel parent is widespread, it is not undisputed; neither the word nor whom should be included within it. The program Språket (The Language) on the Swedish public radio recently had a discussion about the word. One listener had a question about an alternative word, since she thought angel parent was 'too religious' Professor Andersson, the radio expert, had not heard of any synonym and just verified the need and the wide usage of angel parent on the Internet (Språket 2009).

In discussions on the Web about who should be included (for example in parental communities), there is usually an inclusive view regarding those who have lost older children. The word angel parent is not commonly used then but seems accepted on the occasions that it is used. On the other hand, for parents who have lost children very early during pregnancy, it seems different. Some get provoked when parents say they 'lost a child' in the 10th pregnancy week. They argue that it is such a different thing than losing a child late in the pregnancy and that the same word should not be used. However, there are also some who have had a late miscarriage but who do not want to be called angel parents, as the radio listener above also stated.

These discussions inevitably raise questions about 'measuring' grief. Is grief the same, or 'as big' after losing a child to early miscarriage in comparison to losing a child that has lived for many weeks or months? On a general level, one can see that the later in the pregnancy a child is lost, especially if the child lives, the more the parents can interact with the child. That could be one sign of a difference and a way to measure attachment as a correlation to grief. On the other hand, the individual differences are large. For some, the experiences, as could be seen in reactions, behaviour, and comments, are of a similar kind, independent of when the loss takes place. Even an early miscarriage can evoke very strong feeling.

Regardless of these distinctions it is possible to state that the introduction of the concepts angel babies and parents of angels have made a group identification possible, which in itself seems to be important.

Facilitated Communication and a Virtual Community

Even if the nursing and medical care for the parents of a stillborn has improved radically during the last fifteen years, it is doubtful if the reactions of family, friends, and others have changed significantly. Many parents are a witness of silence, avoidance, and isolation. In this aspect, the Internet has come to play an enormous role. The Web facilitates information search and sharing, as well as communication with persons who do not recoil from conversations regarding the experiences of grief.

Today, it is easy to get into contact with others through open communities and closed groups for parents who have lost children. Parents turn to these places, sometimes just a few days after the child is born, sometimes several months later when ordinary life never seems to come back. Within minutes, they can get support and sympathy as well as suggestions for whatever they wonder.

Internet communities are easily accessible. The support groups that meet IRL (in real life) are often concentrated in bigger cities, and with the (fortunately) low infant mortality in a partly sparsely populated country such as Sweden, the Internet makes a real difference. Other studies have shown that support groups on the Internet function both for information support and for emotional support (Capitulo 2004, Malik and Coulson 2008, Coursaris and Liu 2009). Interacting with others in virtual communication has psychosocial benefits. Also, Web memorials have positive benefits, linking the bereaved with the dead as well as with others (Roberts 2004).

One feature of the Web is the possibility to only reveal part of one's identity. On open discussion groups, the first contact is sometimes taken anonymously and then later switches to the use of nicknames. Even in face-to-face groups (such as Alcoholics Anonymous), it is possible to just share as much as one wants about oneself; it is easier to be anonymous on the Web, which might be important in the beginning. Later, and especially in closed support groups, people in Internet groups tend to be very intimate with one another.

Another aspect of the Internet is the support from unknown people. Reading through guest books on Web memorial sites, it is obvious that much acknowledgment can be received from unknown persons who do not necessarily have their own experience of grief but who have read the Web page. Many messages have the form of 'I'm really sorry for what happened to you,' or, 'I have read about your wonderful daughter and I'm thinking of you.' These comments accentuate and acknowledge the grief of the parents and the stillborn as a child from others' view point, which is highly valued, even if communication with other grieving parents is more supportive (Roberts 2006). It is a marking of the grieving parents' identity, quite different from the experiences of friends shifting sidewalks when meeting them.

Photographs

One hundred years ago, around the beginning of 1900, it was not unusual to take pictures of dead persons, including small babies. This was in the early times of photography, and sometimes these pictures are arranged with the whole family standing around the coffin. A couple of decades later, the custom of post-mortem photography disappeared (Åhrén Snickare 2002).

During the last twenty to thirty years the trend has reversed in that parents are encouraged to hold the child but also to take pictures, often by a professional photographer (Rådestad et al. 1996, Godel 2007). With the photographs in hands comes the question what to do with them. While some put them in a drawer or personal photo album, it is also clear from conversations on the Web that many parents use the photographs more actively. They show them to others in the same way as proud parents to living children show their children. One mother writes that she first wondered what she should do with the picture, but then she brought it to her workplace to keep it there as her colleagues had pictures of their children. These kinds of pictures have several social functions – outward, showing colleagues the family identity, and inward, reminding the person about the child and creating a link between the child and the parent. It is a way of 'reconstructing, reinforcing and continuing the biography of the family' (Godel 2007: 259).

On the Internet, photographs of stillborn babies are commonly used on Web memorial pages (Hagström 2006, Godel 2007). Photographs of children in their bed and in the arms of the mother and father appear on many memorial sites.

Even if memorial sites for children born in the midst of pregnancy are unusual, it is possible to find those with photographs of children born in the 20th to 22nd pregnancy week.

Photographs of dead children arouse many thoughts and feelings, and sometimes there are quite strong reactions to them, including discussions about whether they ought to be published on a public space like the Internet (Davidsson Bremborg 2008). These debates show, not withstanding, that such images now have a place in the homes of grieving parents and on the Internet.

Memorialization

The main official ritual for a stillborn is the funeral. Today, almost all parents want a funeral for their stillborn child. Since the new liturgical handbook was published in 1986 the Church of Sweden (a Lutheran Church) has a special funeral ritual for stillborn babies (or children who have died young), which could be seen as a recognition of the stillborn, different from how the Catholic Church has reacted until recently (Garattini 2007, Peelen 2009). Stillborn babies cannot be baptized according to the dogma of the Church, though there is often a name-giving ritual with a blessing led by the hospital chaplaincy.

However, ritualization after death extends beyond the funeral. It is a question of memorialization in a broader sense. In the home, parents create their own memorial place, on a shelf or a table, with candles, photographs, and other mementos. Another kind of ritualization takes place by the grave, especially on certain memorial days (Klass 1999, Francis et al. 2000) (also see Woodthorpe, this volume). These memorial rituals are performed privately and with a personal character. However, they are no longer private in the sense of being untold in the public arena. For example, on memorial sites, parents write about what they are doing on anniversary days: giving birthday presents to the child, talking to the child, wishing him or her a nice day, and eating a birthday cake at home or by the grave.

One special memorial ritual for the stillborn is the blowing of bubbles at the grave site. It is a ritual quite often mentioned on the Swedish sites, but I have also found it on pages from other countries. Among bereaved parents, this is an acknowledged ritual. The origin of the rite is unknown to me, and outside the group, I would regard it as completely unfamiliar. The symbolic thoughts behind the ritual, as described, are interesting. The bubbles lifting toward the sky are seen as links to the child, at the same time as they represent a ‘children’s thing,’ something that parents had hoped their child would one day be able to do.

So far, I have only mentioned the Internet as a communication arena for talking about ritualization, but there are also rituals that can be performed on the Internet. The clearest example is the lighting of virtual candles. Web sites for this ritual opened after catastrophes like 9/11 in 2001, the Indian Ocean tsunami in 2004, and the murder of the foreign minister Anna Lindh in Sweden in 2003. Today, there are lots of Web sites for lighting a candle for someone missing, often with a possibility to write a short message underneath, and of course, there are some also for stillborn babies.

An alternative to the candles is the lighting of a star that one family has on their memorial site for their son (www.wennerstrand.se/william/stjarnhimmel.php). On the dark sky, 279 stars are shining, stars that have been 'lit' online during the last 5 years. The stars make a strong impression. Compared with the candles accompanied with the message where the written words tend to be in focus, the stars shine not only individually but collectively as well. The text messages appear when the cursor hovers over the stars.

Concluding Remarks

For almost seven years, I have followed discussions and events on the Internet regarding stillborn children. It started with an interest in how death is described in the public sphere. Over time, I have seen that the Internet has been revolutionary for bereaved parents. The possibilities for accessing information about stillbirth and grief have increased radically, and the chances to get in contact with parents with similar experiences have become a lot easier. Many parents of stillborn babies experience a silence and void after the death, and thus, the communicative aspect of the Internet is of major importance. However, in some ways, the development has not been as strong as I thought it would be. For example, Web memorials have not increased significantly. I find fewer today than I expected a few years ago. Maybe parents are more aware of the risks that could follow with a home page: photographs can be copied and used on other sites, and critical comments about what they do, think, and say can appear, either in the guest book or (which is more probable) on other sites. Neither is the role of the Internet for the grief undisputed. However, there will always be a diversity of ways to grieve. Some will find the Internet a help, others not.

Norms and values concerning grief have impact on norms regarding ritualization; when norms changes, so do the rituals. As official religion loses its authority, ritualization takes on new forms. These new rituals are private and personal but formed by the collective in narratives. The private rituals seem to need affirmation from others, a negotiation, and reconstruction forming the norms and values of ritualization.

The Internet and the new ways of grief work together. In a changing situation, although individualized and personal, there is still a need for a social context and an endorsement of values, norms, and identities. Consequently, narrative communication on the Internet works as an affirmation in an unstable situation. This is true not only for the psychophysical and emotional situation of grief but also for the spiritual and ritual situation. With a more open discourses of grief following stillbirth, the discourse of ritualization has changed. Where many used to feel isolated, with little support from the caregivers and people around them, there was also a ritual void. Grief following stillbirth could be an isolated and silent experience. If private memorial rituals existed, they were not talked about or visible to others. Today, emotional feelings of grief are shared as well as stories about memorial ritualization. These stories 'normalize' ritualization behaviour, changing norms about what can be done and what is considered appropriate grief behaviour. The private ritual gets a collective normative role by its visibility on the Internet.

Epilogue

A month after the first posted message that appeared at the beginning of this chapter, the mother wrote again about the memorial party, which came to include a memorialization ritual by the grave. With the invitation, she had sent a piece of paper on which guests could write a message to her daughter and leave at the grave. To her surprise, the guests took part in the ritual, not only physically but also by acknowledging the identity of her child:

> I was really pleased. The relatives wrote about how they were related to NN, and that is very unusual. I was shocked when I saw it … They wrote on the piece of paper I had given them, and then finished with 'grandpa/aunt/grandma' + their name. That really warmed the cockles of my heart!

References

Åhrén Snickare, E. 2002. *Döden, kroppen och moderniteten*. Stockholm: Carlsson.

Andersson Wretmark, A. 1993. *Perinatal Death as a Pastoral Problem*. Stockholm: Almqvist & Wiksell.

Bäckström, A., Edgardh Beckman., N. and Pettersson, P. 2004. *Religious Change in Northern Europe: The Case of Sweden*. Stockholm: Verbum.

Capitulo, K.L. 2004. Perinatal grief online. *American Journal of Maternal Child Nursing*, 29(5), 305-311.

Castells, M. 2001. *The Internet Galaxy: Reflexions on the Internet, Business and Society*. Oxford: Oxford University Press.

Coursaris, C.K. and Liu, M. 2009. An analysis of social support exchanges in online HIV/AIDS self-help groups. *Computers in Human Behavior*, 25(4), 911-918.

Davie, G. 1994. *Religion in Britain since 1945: Believing without Belonging*. Oxford: Blackwell.

Davies, D.J. 1997. *Death, Ritual and Belief: The Rhetoric of Funerary Rites*. London: Cassell.

Davidsson Bremborg, A. 2009. Dead bodies on the Internet, in *Making Sense of Death, Dying and Bereavement: An Anthology*, edited by S. Earle, C. Bartholomew and C. Komaromy. London: Sage, 74-7.

Francis, D., Kellaher, L. and Neophytou, G. 2000. Sustaining cemeteries: the user perspective. *Mortality*, 5(1), 35-54.

Garattini, C. 2008. Creating memories: material culture and infantile death in contemporary Ireland. *Mortality*, 12(2), 193-206.

Giddens, A. 1991. *Modernity and self-identity: self and society in the late modern age*. Cambridge: Polity Press.

Godel, M. 2007. Images of stillbirth: memory, mourning and memorial. *Visual Studies*, 22(3), 253-269.

Grout, L. and Romanoff, B. 2000. The myth of the replacement child: parent stories and practices after perinatal death. *Death Studies*, 24(2), 93-113.

Hagström, C., 2006. *Berättelser om* änglabarn. *Minnessidor på Internet* [Stories about angel children. Memorial sites on the Internet], in HEX001 Virtualiteter: sex essäer, edited by R. Willim. Lund: Humanistiska fakulteten Lunds universitet.

Hallam, E., Hockey, J. and Howarth, G. 1999. *Beyond the Body: Death and Social Identity*. London: Routledge.

Hallam, E. and Hockey, J. 2001. *Death, Memory & Material Culture*. Oxford: Berg.

Hamberg, E.M. 2003. Christendom in decline: the Swedish case, in *The Decline of Christendom in Western Europe*, 1750-2000, edited by H. McLeod and W. Ustort. Cambridge: Cambridge University Press, 47-62.

Heelas, P. and Woodhead, L. 2005. *Why Religion is Giving Way to Spirituality*. Malden, Mass.: Blackwell.

Klass, D. 1999. *The Spiritual Lives of Bereaved Parents* (Series in Death, Dying, and Bereavement). Philadelphia, PA: Brunner/Mazel, Taylor & Francis.

Lagrådsremiss. 2008. *Samordningsnummer och anmälan av dödfödd m.m.* Stockholm 24 januari. Available from: http://www.regeringen.se/sb/d/10163/a/96619 [accessed 25 November 2011].

Lundqvist, A.N. 1998. Neonatal death and parents' grief – experiences, behaviour and attitudes of Swedish nurses. *Scandinavian Journal Caring Sciences*, 12(4), 246-250.

Malik, S.H. and Coulson, N.S. 2008. Computer-mediated infertility support groups: An exploratory study of online experiences. *Patient Education and Counseling*, 73(1), 105-113.

Peelen, J. 2009. Reversing the past: Monuments for stillborn children. *Mortality*, 14(2), 173-186.

Rådestad, I. 1999. *When a Meeting is also Farewell: Coping with a Stillbirth or Neonatal Death*. Hale: Books for Midwives.

Rådestad, I., Nordin, C., Steineck, G. and Sjögren, B. 1996. Stillbirth is no longer managed as a nonevent: A nationwide study in Sweden. *Birth*, 23(4), 209-215.

Riches, G. and Dawson, P. 1998. Lost children, living memories: the role of photographs in processes of grief and adjustment among bereaved parent. *Death Studies*, 22(2), 121-140.

Roberts, P. 2004. The Living and the Dead. Community in the Virtual Cemetery. *Omega*, 49(1), 57-76.

Roberts, P. 2006. From My Space to Our Space: The Functions of Web Memorials in Bereavement. *The Forum*, 32(4), 1-4. Association for Death Education and Counseling.

Säflund, K. 2003. *An analysis of parents' experiences and the caregivers' role following the birth of a stillborn child.* Unpublished PhD Thesis. Stockholm, Sweden.

SAOL, 2006. *Svenska akademiens ordlista* över *svenska språket.* 13th ed. Stockholm: Svenska akademien.

SCB. 2009. *Statistikdatabasen. Datoranvändning bland privatpersoner 16-74* år *efter kön,* ålder *och hur ofta man använt persondator (urvalsundersökning)*. År 2003-2008. [Online]. Available at: www.scb.se (accessed: 25 November 2011).

SFS. 1991:481. *Folkbokföringslag* (National civil registration law).

SFS 2008:207. *Lag om* ändring *i folkbokföringslagen.*

Språket, *Sveriges radio* (Swedish Radio). 2009. [Online]. Available at: <http://www.sr.se/laddahem/podradio/SR_p1_spraket_090303020058.mp3> (accessed: 25 November 2011).

Walter, T. 1996. A new model of grief: bereavement and biography. *Mortality*, 1(1), 7-25.

World Health Organization (WHO). 1992. *International statistical classification of diseases and related health problems. ICD-10.* Geneva: World Health Organization. [Online]. Available at: http://libris.kb.se/bib/9888482;jsessionid=5188E253A4CD6A014BB7DE9437BCCFDA (accessed: 25 November 2011).

Chapter 13

'As If She Never Existed': Changing Understandings of Perinatal Loss in Australia in the Twentieth and Early Twenty-First Century

Susannah Thompson

In May 1967, two women shared a room in a small private maternity hospital in Perth, Western Australia. Their room was situated next door to the nursery, where both women could hear the busyness of the nurses and the cries of newborn babies. These women were strangers to each other, but they shared a sad bond as mothers. One, a young unmarried woman, was waiting to give birth to a baby who would then be relinquished for adoption, despite her own misgivings. The other woman, Audrey, was recuperating after giving birth to a stillborn baby, her third child. When I asked Audrey what she remembered of her time spent in the hospital, she recalled that her baby was 'whisked away' and that she spent the next week recovering from a postnatal infection whilst the nurses 'tiptoed around' her. She then left the hospital without any knowledge as to why her baby had died, or where his remains had been buried. However, her dominant memory of this period is particularly poignant: 'We [both] could hear the crying [of babies]. That's all I remember of the hospital' (Thompson 2008).

Despite advancements in medical knowledge of foetal development and the decline in infant mortality, miscarriage, stillbirth and neonatal death remain all-too common events in many Australian women's (and their families') lives. Recent statistics estimate as many as 1 in 4 pregnancies end in miscarriage and over 10 in 100 ends in stillbirth or neonatal death in Australia (Australia's Mothers and Babies 2004, National Perinatal Statistics Unit, Australian Institute of Health and Welfare, Sydney, 2006). In spite of this frequency, perinatal loss has been largely neglected in historical scholarship. My doctoral research was an attempt to rectify this lacuna; my thesis charted the wide range of socially constructed meanings of pregnancy loss in twentieth century Australia and in doing so, sought to analyse changing understandings of pregnancy loss over time (Thompson 2008). A crucial component of this research was an oral history project: I interviewed some 30 women who had experienced some form of pregnancy loss. The oldest participant was 90 at the time of the interview in 2005; she had experienced the stillbirth of her first child in 1940. These oral history interviews were then analysed against the socio-historical context of pregnancy loss in Australia, and gave rich insight into how a group of Australian women understood their particular experience of loss at a particular point in time. Although oral history, like any other single source, cannot paint a complete picture, its usefulness lies in its ability to reveal the ways in which an individual has sought to make sense of an incident in their life (Thompson 2010).

Pregnancy Loss Prior to the Medicalization of Childbirth

At the turn of the nineteenth and twentieth centuries, the ending of a pregnancy through miscarriage or perinatal death was an event of great regularity, and the risks to both mother and child posed by childbirth were ever-present concerns. A lack of knowledge of infection during childbirth proved fatal for many Australian women and their babies, whilst poor living conditions in cities led to large outbreaks of infectious diseases such as gastro-enteritis, pneumonia, diphtheria and tuberculosis as well as a high incidence of weanling diarrhoea, making infancy a particularly dangerous period of life (Durey 1982). In the period between 1870 and 1914, 1495 stillbirths (often confused in the record with premature birth) and 5693 infant deaths were recorded in the small city of Perth, Western Australia alone (Durey 1982).

In the late nineteenth century, the fledgling medical profession in Australia scarcely paid heed to infant mortality; pregnancy and childbirth, and its varying outcomes, were largely left to the ministrations of women. Those who attended births in the late nineteenth and early twentieth centuries – usually untrained midwives or peripatetic physicians who delivered the child in the family's home – were often well acquainted with perinatal death. Wilhemina Haub, for example, was a rural Western Australian midwife whose meticulous case notes record several incidents of miscarriage, stillbirth and neonatal death; the latter two usually after a prolonged and obstructed labour. The great distances that Mrs Haub traveled often meant that she arrived after the baby had already been delivered, and her notes reveal that she was not unused to finding that the child had either been born dead or was seriously ill and not expected to survive (Thompson 2008).

Medicalization of Pregnancy and the Discourse of 'Successful' Pregnancy, 1920–1960

Although the late nineteenth century was characterized by a sense of inevitability towards stillbirth and neonatal death amongst the medical profession, several eminent physicians began to argue that 'pregnancy wastage' was largely preventable provided the pregnant body was carefully supervised within the framework of scientific, rational knowledge and, by explicit connection, by the medical profession alone (Thompson 2008). In the late nineteenth and early twentieth centuries numerous Australian physicians recorded their anxieties over the high infant and maternal mortality rates, and a growing subject of discussion in medical journals was the issue of the 'meddlesome and ignorant' midwife and their role in both pregnancy loss and maternal deaths (Willis 1989). Various midwifery registration acts from 1915 to 1920 curtailed the dominance of female birth attendants, culminating with the incorporation of midwifery into nursing in 1928. These events signalled the beginning of medical dominance over pregnancy and childbirth, and the end of childbirth as a matter to be dealt with by women themselves (Willis 1989).

At this time, women's own understandings of their bodies were supplanted by medical discourse, disseminated by the so-called 'wives' handbooks' which were proliferated in the early twentieth century. One handbook, written by an American physician for an Australian audience, admonished women to avoid 'long walks, purgatives, riding in a carriage or on the cars, overwork, worry, fear, fright, sexual intercourse, irritation of the breasts, falls, vomiting [and] convulsions' (Rossiter 1913: 455) whilst another handbook urged women to be 'enlightened [through medical advice] or loss of life to her unborn babe … will, in all probability be the penalties of her ignorance' (Allen and McGregor 1896: 187).

In discrediting women's knowledge and understandings of their pregnant bodies, the medical profession claimed authority to speak about pregnancy and childbirth. For much of the twentieth century, medical discourse inscribed the unborn baby as essentially 'unknown' and 'unknowable' – and therefore replaceable. This led to the prevailing belief that, whilst perinatal loss was a 'sad event', any grief following this event would be resolved by having another baby. This prescription to loss was also part of the cultural expectation that women's 'natural' roles were that of wife and mother, and the act of having subsequent children signified a bereaved woman's willingness to resume 'normal' life by fulfilling her rightful place in Australian society (Thompson 2008).

In the regimented environment of the post-war maternity hospital, principally organized towards the care of live babies and their mothers, the prevailing view was that women should be shielded from the experience of perinatal loss (Curtis 2000). Medical discourse held women as fixed to nature and prone to emotional instability – notions which were reinforced by and reproduced within the cultural shifts towards repressed sorrow after death in the early twentieth century (Jalland 2006). An underlying motivation behind both the removal of the deceased baby's body and the practise of sedating women after a stillbirth was the fear that bereaved mothers would become hysterical and exhibit an 'inappropriate' or 'excessive' emotional response (Thompson 2008). Furthermore, the medical profession itself was dominated by an expectation of emotional aloofness; empathy was scorned as an irrational response, although evidence suggests that some medical professionals found this to be a difficult burden to bear (McCalman 1996; Reiger 2000). Lorna Lloyd Green, a resident at the Royal Women's Hospital in Melbourne in the 1940s, recalled feeling distressed by the brisk and detached response of male obstetricians who dismissed the possibility of any emotional ramifications after a stillbirth or neonatal death:

> What used to worry me no end … especially one obstetrician was: I would say – 'it's just terrible that she's lost that baby, we should have been able to do something about it'. And he'd reply, 'She'll have another'. And I would get mad – 'How do you know that she'll have another? We have no idea that she will have another'. Psychologically and physically there was everything against her (McCalman 1996: 200).

Bereaved mothers, then, were often regarded as anomalies and the unwelcome reminder of a 'failed' birth. Sometimes placed out of sight down a far corridor, at other times, placed back on the maternity ward, those women who miscarried or whose babies died shortly before or after birth presented somewhat of a conundrum for hospital staff. Most of the older women interviewed for this research recalled that they were often sedated after the death of their baby; their babies were 'whisked away' after delivery without the mother catching a glimpse of the body, and they were usually excluded from any burial arrangements and rarely were given any detailed information as to why their baby had died. In describing the attitude of the nurses at the hospital where she delivered her first child, Barbara commented that after her daughter was stillborn at term, 'it was as though she never existed, really, to me. Because I had nothing' (Thompson 2008: 110).

The common practice of placing bereaved women back onto shared maternity wards is indicative of the stoicism expected of women after perinatal loss. Rayma, for example, was placed back on a general postnatal ward after her twin sons were stillborn: 'afterwards they put me into a ward with nursing mothers. That was hard' (Thompson 2008: 116). Iris remembered that upon her admittance to hospital she was initially accommodated in the labour ward in a four-bed room with a woman who was waiting to deliver her deceased baby, whilst Iris – whose baby was still alive at this point – herself waited for labour to begin: 'I sort of said, 'when's yours due?' Because mine was still to come, but the others had had theirs – it was a four-bed, I think. And she just sat there and said, "I've got to wait till it comes. It's dead now"' (Thompson 2008: 116).

Reinforcing the distant approach to obstetrics and gynaecology were the sheer logistical problems facing many maternity wards around Australia during the post-war 'baby boom'. Whilst individual doctors and nurses may have sought to pay more attention to pregnant mothers and bereaved mothers alike, the nature of working in a maternity hospital during this period was likely to be a significant obstacle. Kerreen Reiger (2000) notes that 'post-war labour wards were crowded, noisy, and understaffed' and these constraints meant 'little time for individual attention and the general authoritarianism of hospital routine was unquestioned'. One woman, Margaret, recalled being left to her 'own devices' whilst she waited in hospital for her labour to begin. The nurses were busy preparing for the hospital fête, and, according to Margaret, 'they just sort of didn't take much notice of me, and I can remember walking all the way down from the hospital right down to the river, having a lovely walk down' (Thompson 2008: 112).

Certainly some women were treated with kindness and gentleness despite the hustle and bustle of the post-war maternity ward; Iris, for example was granted an unusual request because of, she believes, her friendship with the sister of one of the nurses. Although she had not been permitted to view her daughter's body, Iris requested that she be able to hold someone else's baby for a while 'because everything in you just wants to do that'. The request was met with some consternation, but it was eventually granted, to Iris' pleasure. Iris recalled that:

> There was a bit of a turmoil amongst the staff, because I'd asked, and whose baby would it be, that sort of thing. And anyway somehow they agreed, went to the women and asked for a volunteer, I don't know how it happened but the next thing someone brought in – not the mother, a nurse, brought in a little baby, and I just had a hold and a little cuddle and then handed it back, of course. But if felt, sort of, expressed something from within me [but] of course it couldn't go on and on (Thompson 2008: 113).

The practice of 'shielding' women from the experience of perinatal loss was not restricted to the hospital setting. A significant cultural shift of the early twentieth century had been a repressing of public rituals of mourning. The cumulative effects of the two world wars in less than thirty years had led to an expectation that grief was a private affair and that public display of grief was unseemly and indulgent (Jalland 2006). Despite the expectation that the expression of grief should remain private, some women did attempt to share their grief with family and friends, but found that their loss was rejected. They concluded that they had been unwise to share their feelings, and that their grief should be internalized and remain a private affair. Ivy, for example, ventured to tell some close friends that she and her husband had named the child, but was deeply hurt when the couple openly articulated their opinion that 'oh they've named the baby – that's a bit stupid!' After hearing this callous remark, Ivy determined that she 'wouldn't talk about it anymore' – acknowledging that this was how she perceived what was expected of her anyway: 'We never discussed it. Now, everything is discussed, but then we never discussed anything. You never asked – well I didn't' (Thompson 2008: 130).

Towards a More Open Expression of Grief after Perinatal Loss, 1970– 1990

The late 1960s saw a growing recognition that perhaps the stoic response of former generations was not necessarily beneficial; the expression of grief, it was argued, could be healing and appropriate. The work of Elisabeth Kübler-Ross (1970) and John Bowlby (1969), on the stages of grief and the mother-infant bond respectively, paved the way for studies which focused specifically on the experience of losing an unborn child. In Australia, two studies in particular marked a significant shift in the way that perinatal loss was understood. In 1970, Professor Patrick Giles at King Edward Memorial Hospital for Women (KEMH) in Western Australia proffered his cautious findings that a woman might experience feelings of grief after a perinatal loss (Giles 1970). The 1986 work of psychologist Margaret Nicol, also at KEMH, took this one step further, when she argued that the loss of a baby could be as psychologically influential as the loss of a spouse (Nicol 1984). These studies, along with other research being conducted in British and American institutions, would gradually alter the understanding that the unborn child was essentially 'unknowable' and that grief after perinatal loss was likely to be minimal.

By the 1970s the conservative trust in the medical profession's authority that so marked many prior decades was being questioned, particularly with regard to the surveillance and supervision of women's bodies during pregnancy and childbirth. The growing homebirth movement was testament to this dissatisfaction, as more and more women demanded that their needs and desires in labour and childbirth be considered. Women began to choose homebirth in order to 'reclaim' control over their bodies; to demand that they be able to give birth to their children without routine use of analgesia and other interventions such as episiotomy; and for the opportunity to be close to their child immediately after birth and for their partner to be able to play a significant role in the birth – features which were not likely to be a part of the experience of giving birth before this period (Reiger 2000).

This challenge to conservative ideas of the treatment of labour and childbirth, and the emerging studies on grief reactions after perinatal loss would gradually change hospital practice with regards to perinatal loss. Driven by the ideals of feminism, midwives and other allied-health professionals, such as social workers, challenged the masculinist medical discourse which constructed the body in purely physiological terms, and they sought to raise awareness of the fact that women, as important consumers of hospital services, were not being served well (Thompson 2007b). Nursing education in the past had emphasized an aloof approach to patients and had placed little, if any, emphasis on individuality, but the late 1970s and early 1980s marked a new trend in nursing and midwifery care. In 1978, the National Body of Midwives was formed, and through this association there were efforts to educate nurses and midwives of the need to treat all patients with compassion and dignity – to treat the 'whole person', not just the physical condition. During the early 1980s, midwives began to take an interest in the emerging ideas of grief and loss and professional development seminars were held at both national and state levels to help educate those who were involved in the care of dying patients, including babies. The 'Death and Dying Workshop' at Monash University in Melbourne in September 1980, for example, was intended for 'professional staff and others whose work involves them with the dying and bereaved and those coping with loss', and speakers included Des Tobin, an experienced funeral director, and Patricia Harrison, a lecturer in obstetrics and gynaecology at the University of Melbourne (Thompson 2008) Similarly, the Midwives Annual City Seminar for

1981 focused solely on perinatal death and the midwife's role and involvement in this event (Thompson 2008).

At the Royal Women's Hospital in Melbourne and King Edward Memorial Hospital for Women in Perth, some social workers and midwives, along with a few obstetricians, spearheaded the push to change the way that women were treated when they came to hospital to give birth. Coupled with the emerging literature on the psychosocial needs of pregnant women, as well as the embracing of feminism, was the fact that the late 1970s and early 1980s heralded a major shift in community attitudes towards ex-nuptial birth. In the decades prior to the 1970s, most social workers were preoccupied with adoption issues, but as single motherhood became more socially acceptable and financially viable, social workers were able to turn their focus to other needs within the hospital (McCalman 1996). Although allied health professionals were no doubt affected by theorists of grief and loss, many were keen to find ways to actually implement theory and a crucial part of this became listening to parents themselves (Thompson 2007a). This was of course a radical step, moving from the authoritative voice of the medical profession, who held themselves responsible for disseminating medical knowledge and information, towards a parent–focused approach that sought to value the needs and desires of the patient, and privileged patients' dignity (McCalman 1996). For perhaps the first time, health professionals sought the wisdom of bereaved parents in seeking to understand what parents felt they wanted and needed after the death of their baby. Other Australian health professionals, such as Peter Barr, an obstetrician, and his wife, social worker Deborah de Wilde, echoed the importance of recognising the individual nature of grief saying that 'each person experiences of expresses his or her grief differently according to a number of different factors including past childhood and adolescent experiences and the meaning and significance attached to the person who died' (Barr and de Wilde 1987).

In the area of perinatal death, most early practical change grew out of the intensive care nursery, and was later extended to the care of women whose babies were stillborn or miscarried. The pioneering work of prominent American physicians Klaus, Slyter and Kennel (1970) had opened the door for women to be granted contact with their dying or critically ill newborns and it was increasingly understood that this could produce beneficial results rather than irrevocably harm the woman, as had been believed for many years (Helmrath and Steinitz 1978). In the KEMH Neonatal Intensive Care Unit, for example, two social workers out of a complete staff of four were responsible for psychosocial care of parents of preterm infants, which grew to encompass the care of parents whose babies died. A social worker at the hospital remembered that she and a few other nurses would 'orchestrate it a little bit if you like, as in, go to a quiet room, sit with the people, help the relatives, what are we going to do with the children, with grandma, bring cups of tea, tissues, all that sort of stuff' (Thompson 2008: 149). It is interesting to note that this was the same trajectory for similar bereaved parents' groups in the United States, which are discussed in more detail by Linda Layne (2006). Clearly, the Australian context was greatly influenced by trends in the United States and Britain.

A significant agent for change at this time was parents themselves. Recent trends in the community had meant that hospital care was gradually growing more patient-focused and listening to parents' needs was a significant step towards changing ways of supporting women who had lost a baby (Milliken 1978). The manifestation of listening to parents, at KEMH at least, coupled with the enthusiasm of some staff for the ideals of a supportive 'sisterhood', was the birth of several support groups. At KEMH in 1980, recalled social worker Libby Lloyd:

> One of the things that I did was to establish a self-help group called PIPA – Preterm Infant Parents' Association – and after a little while of those gatherings, we made a video of people talking about their experiences and so on, [and] there came a parent who said, 'well I had a prem., but it died and I need help now for its dying', and then another who said 'I had a prem., but it was to do with IVF', so we started Concern for the Infertile, and then we started off SANDS. So in one glorious year there were three of these groups running (Thompson 2008: 150)

All but Support After Neonatal Death [SANDS] faded over time, but the recognition that women would most likely need support after the death of a baby – and that women could draw great support from each other – was an idea that persisted. In Australian hospitals SANDS and later, other support groups for bereaved parents, acted as important players in changing attitudes towards perinatal death as well as provided a sort of haven for parents once they had left the hospital (Thompson 2007c).

The emerging theories of grief and loss significantly undermined the dominant understanding of pregnancy loss as a sad, but easily forgotten, event in a woman's life; nonetheless it would be some time before the early work of some social workers and midwives was recognized as official hospital policy. Alice Lovell (1983) observed of the British context in the early 1980s that 'maternity units are geared to the production of live babies. When this goes wrong, there is the … problem of what do with the maternity patient – is she a patient?' It can be assumed that this was often the case in Australian hospitals. For example, after the stillbirth of her daughter, Kaye was aware that her baby had died before labour started, and remembers feeling that she did not quite 'fit' as a maternity patient: 'One nurse … made a few heartless comments during labour. I'm sure she was busy but made a comment to another nurse that it was a 'waste of time' bringing a crib into the delivery suite as it wouldn't be needed. I didn't need to hear this – it was the reality of the situation but a little tactless I felt' (Thompson 2008: 166).

Nonetheless, by the 1990s it was widely accepted that the practice of 'protection' was not an appropriate way of managing perinatal death. Coupled with this was a new openness towards death in many parts of Australian society. Formalized hospital policies at KEMH in WA and RWH in Victoria reflected the construction of perinatal death as an event of great significance in a woman's life.

The rejection of the practice of 'protection' in favour of assisting women to form attachments with their deceased babies and the shift away from hospital disposal or mass burial towards individual burial rituals, for example, give insight into the radical changes to the management of perinatal loss and the reinscribing of the deceased baby as eminently 'knowable' and irreplaceable. By the last decade of the twentieth century it was progressively more accepted by many health care professionals, and particularly social workers and midwives, that many parents understood their stillborn baby or deceased infant to a precious member of the family despite having not lived outside the womb, or for just a short time, and some hospitals around the country, including King Edward Memorial Hospital in Perth and the Royal Women's Hospital in Melbourne, had begun to respond to this knowledge by implementing routines that were geared towards caring for bereaved women and their families (Thompson 2007a).

At KEMH, for example, in response to the need to educate all staff who came into contact with bereaved parents, the late 1980s had seen the introduction of the 'teardrop programme' at maternity hospitals in Western Australia. An initiative of SANDS (Western Australia) this involved the placing of small teardrop shaped stickers on the doors of rooms accommodating bereaved women, a move designed to alert all staff from gynaecologists to ward stewards as to the need for sensitivity and diplomacy (Thompson 2008). The Grief Kit was also a significant creation at KEMH, developed by SANDS and KEMH social workers, and which would later be used complete or modified by most major hospitals around the country. The concept of the Grief Kits was not restricted to the Australian context; Layne (2000) has also noted the use of artefacts in making memories after loss in the United States of America. The Grief Kits designed by SANDS (WA) aimed to help parents create a tangible record of their baby: a way of honouring the memory of the stillborn or deceased baby where little tangible evidence existed. Underpinning the kit's development was the belief that each stillborn or deceased newborn child was, most often, perceived to be a valued member of a family and worthy of such validation. The kits also contained several leaflets on the grieving process and, some time later, physiological issues such as milk suppression and how to cope with 'after pains' (Thompson 2007c).

Prenatal Testing and the 'Window to the Womb': Renewing the Discourse of 'Successful' Pregnancy, 1990–present

Towards the end of the twentieth century, however, these changing constructions of pregnancy loss were problematized with the medical profession's increased ability to 'screen' the foetal body for 'imperfection'. The Western Australian Department of Health Prenatal Screening and Diagnosis Study (2001) found that two-thirds of women surveyed had at least one ultrasound during pregnancy, and one-third had a maternal serum screening. The rise of prenatal screening and the expectation that women should strive for reproductive 'perfection' has increasingly produced a cultural expectation that women can, and should, control their behaviours and bodies to produce trouble-free pregnancies and deliveries.

The prescriptions for a normal, healthy birth have cultivated a 'moral component' of pregnancy which has led to an expectation that if women manage their pregnancy appropriately, they will be rewarded with a healthy baby (Crouch and Manderson 1993). The corollary of this expectation is the implication that women have been to blame if their baby died. In the best-selling Australian edition of *What to Expect when you're Expecting*, the authors of the comprehensive pregnancy advice manual respond to the statement that 'I had the perfect first baby … I can't shake the fear that I won't be so lucky this time' with the reassurance that 'your chances of hitting the jackpot again are excellent. A mother who has had a perfect baby isn't only likely to win again, her odds are better than they were before she had a successful pregnancy under her belt' (Eisenberg et al 1996: 24). The strong implication is, of course, that women who have had a previously 'imperfect' baby have not 'won' but have lost in their quest for the perfect baby; furthermore, this loss has been caused in some way by their failure to control their pregnancy adequately. In the late twentieth century, the rise of prenatal screening has wrought a re-emergence of ideas of 'appropriate' maternal behaviours, potentially leading to stigmatization for those women whose experiences of expectant and early motherhood fall short of these ideals.

Pregnancy loss has been understood in a range of ways by different groups over the past century, and beyond, in Australia. At the turn of the century, alarm was mounting over the shockingly high maternal and infant mortality rates, and untrained and unregistered birth attendants were seen as largely culpable for pregnancy loss. The medicalization of childbirth in the early twentieth century, with its expectation of medically-supervised pregnancy and birth, supplanted the earlier tradition of women tending to pregnancy and childbirth; it also displaced women's own understandings of their pregnant body and by extension, pregnancy loss. For much of the twentieth century, it was widely believed that pregnancy loss was an event that would be soon forgotten, particularly if women were 'shielded' from any grief reactions. Oral history testimony gives insight into the ways in which this was manifest: many women were not given the opportunity to see their deceased babies, or were told little as to why their babies had died. Moreover, cultural attitudes towards death in post-war Australia compounded the silence surrounding pregnancy loss, with the prevailing expectation that repressed sorrow was the appropriate response to grief. Cultural shifts in the 1970s and 1980s, inspired by international trends, led to a more patient-centred understanding of pregnancy and childbirth in general, and pregnancy loss in particular. In the last two decades of the twentieth century, it was more widely understood, at least within the hospital setting, that pregnancy loss was a potentially devastating event. The increasingly routine use of prenatal testing in the twenty-first century has problematized meanings of pregnancy loss in Australia, by cultivating the expectation that women's behaviours and decisions during pregnancy directly impact the outcome of a pregnancy.

References

AIHW. National Perinatal Statistics Unit, 2006. *Australia's Mothers and Babies 2004*. Australian Institute of Health and Welfare: Sydney.

Barr, P. and de Wilde, D. 1987. *Stillbirth and Newborn Death: Death and Life are the Same Mysteries*. Camperdown, NSW.

Crouch, M. and Manderson, L. 1993. *New Motherhood: Cultural and Personal Transitions in the 1980s*. Yverdon, Switzerland: Gordon and Breach Sciences.

Curtis, P. 2000. Midwives' Attendances at Stillbirths: an oral history account. *Midwifery Digest*, Dec, 526-530.

Damousi, J. 1999. *The Labour of Loss: Mourning, Memory and Wartime Bereavement in Australia*. Cambridge, Melbourne: Cambridge University Press.

Durey, M. 1982. Infant Mortality in Perth, Western Australia, 1870-1914: A preliminary analysis. *Studies in Western Australian History*, 5, 62–71.

Eisenberg, A., Eisenberg Murkoff, H. and Eisenberg Hathaway, S. 1996. *What to Expect When You're Expecting*. Sydney: Angus and Robertson.

Giles, P.F.H. 1970. Reactions of Women to Perinatal Death. *Australian New Zealand Journal of Obstetrics and Gynaecology*, 10, 207-211.

Helmrath, T. and Steinitz, E. 1978. Death of an Infant: Parental Grieving and the Failure of Social Support. *Journal of Family Practice*, 6(4), 790.

Jalland, P. 2006. *Changing Ways of Death in Twentieth Century Australia: War, Medicine and the Funeral Business*. Sydney: University of New South Wales Press.

Kennell, J, Klaus, M. and Slyer, H. 1970. The Mourning Response of Parents to the Death of a Newborn Infant. *New England Journal of Medicine*, 283, 344-349.

Kűbler-Ross, E. 1970. *On Death and Dying*. New York: Macmillan.

Layne, L. 2000. 'He was a Real Baby with Baby Things': A Material Culture Analysis of Personhood and Pregnancy Loss. *Journal of Material Culture*, 5(3), 321-345.

Layne, L. 2003. *Motherhood Lost: A Feminist Account of Pregnancy Loss in America*. New York, London: Routledge.

Layne, L. 2006. Pregnancy and Infant Loss Support: A New Feminist, American, Patient Movement? *Social Science and Medicine* special issue on Patient Organization Movements, 62(3), 602-613.

Lovell, A. 1983. Some questions of identity: late miscarriage, stillbirth and perinatal loss. *Social Science and Medicine*, 17(11), 757-761.

McCalman, J. 1996. *Sex and Suffering: Women's Health and a Women's Hospital: The Royal Women's Hospital Melbourne, 1856-1996*. Carlton, Vic: Melbourne University Press.

Milliken, D. 1978. Changes in the Neonatal Nurse's Role. *Australian Nursing Journal*, 8(4), 30-33 & 40.

Nicol, M. 1984. *The Loss of a Baby: Understanding Maternal Grief*. Sydney: Bantam.

Reiger, K. 2000. *Our Bodies, Our Babies: The Forgotten Women's Movement*. Carlton, Vic.: Melbourne University Press.

Rossiter, F. 1913. *The Practical Guide to Health*. Melbourne: Signs Publishing.

Thompson, S. 2007a. Experimenting with Change: Experiences of miscarriage, stillbirth and neonatal death in Australia in the 1980s. *Journal of Australian Studies (New Talents)*, 67-76.

Thompson, S. 2007b. Out of the stirrups: the impact of childbirth reform and second wave feminism in the 1970s and 1980s on the management of perinatal death. *Birth Issues*, 15(3-4), 83-88.

Thompson, S. 2007c. 'Awakened by angels': personal narratives of perinatal death in the late twentieth century in Western Australia and their impact on hospital policy and programmes. *Studies in Western Australian History*, 25, 166-180.

Thompson, S. 2008. *Birth Pains: Changing Understandings of Miscarriage, Stillbirth and Neonatal Death in Australia in the Twentieth Century*. Unpublished PhD thesis, University of Western Australia.

Thompson, S. 2010. 'I didn't talk to anybody': reflections on researching the history of perinatal loss in Australia. *Studies in Western Australian History*, 26, 163-175.

Western Australian Department of Health. 2001. *Prenatal Screening and Diagnosis Study*.

Willis, E. 1989. *Medical Dominance: the Division of Labour in Australian Health Care*. Sydney: Allen and Unwin.

Chapter 14

Hiding Babies: How Birth Professionals Make Sense of Death and Grief

Jan Bleyen

Ann felt as if her world had turned upside down. In the early days of her midwifery career, she and her colleagues did everything they could to keep a stillborn baby as far away as possible from his or her mother. However, on moving to another ward in the early 1990s, Ann was struck by the way that nurses, doctors and midwives all took the deceased baby to its mum whenever she wanted to see it. Hence in contrast to older procedures with which she had always been familiar, the practice of getting to know the physical features of the stillborn son or daughter was now assumed to be a healthy thing to do.

In my historical contribution here, I do not aim to criticise – or idealise – old routines versus new ones. Rather I want to explore how culture in terms of how people understand the world they live in metaphorically underpins both past and current practices. Therefore, the question I will raise is: how do birth professionals make sense of death and grief through the act of hiding or showing a stillborn child?

Metaphors

The experience of losing a child at birth has received much attention primarily from psychological and action-oriented scholars who focus on the individual griever rather than the social and cultural contexts (see Cecil 1996, Layne 2003) which include professionals' practices and beliefs. This area has been largely neglected by historians.

Nevertheless, it provides a multifaceted topic for the anthropological history of reproduction and endings, the body and emotions, identity and personhood.

In this chapter I draw on open-ended, qualitative interview data from retired and practising Flemish gynaecologists, midwives and pastors in small-scale hospital environments to illustrate how hiding the dead babies' bodies was an act of 'performing' different meanings of death and grief, in a corporal and sensory way.[1]

1 This study was part of my doctoral dissertation conducted at the Subfaculty of History at the Katholieke Universiteit Leuven in Belgium, during my assistantship from

Using metaphors and narrative forms (see Polkinghorne 1988, Riessman 2008) I develop two contrasting and partially historical approaches to everyday clinical practice and meaning-making – a 'distant' and an 'intimate' one. However, following the recent historians' performative turn (Burke 2005: 35), the hiding of stillborn babies is suggested not only to have confirmed specific cultural patterns of meaning and images of the self but also to have generated them. In other words, situated in a historical approach, hiding babies can be analysed as an occasional practice transforming not only the material reality of the ward atmosphere (Edvardsson, Rasmussen and Riessman 2003) and its embodied subjects, but also by the abstract concepts of death and grief.

The answer to the question 'What is death?' is far from universal and the concrete ways of understanding death vary from culture to culture. Furthermore, multiple definitions of death exist within one context because of the various perspectives from which they are acted upon. This is because death belongs not only to human nature but also to the shifting world of cultural meanings and social practices. Hence, ways of conceptualizing death are dynamic and multiple (Bleyen 2009).

I argue that 'death' can only be made present through metaphors: conceptual constructs that are pervasive not only in language but also in thought and practice. This is because the reality of death is simply impossible to imagine. Every statement on death refers to other symbols rather than to an empirical reality. Hence death is conceptualized and acted upon as a process (for example, dying), an instance (for example, the Grim Reaper), a state (for example, the absence of life), or a moment (for example, one's final breath) (see Kellehear 2007). It is only through such metaphors that the idea of death becomes a tangible entity. In other words, defining death requires an act of presentation, rather than one of representation. It is a performative act in as far as each definition of death fixes a specific context and brings forth death in one way or another. Correspondingly, death is defined through metaphors in the social practice of birth professionals (Bleyen 2009). Lakoff and Johnson define a metaphor as a device which is deeply embedded in conceptual thinking and which plays a significant role in providing something intangible with a tangible image or story. Significantly, metaphor stands in for reality (see Sontag 1979 and Hockey, Komaromy and Woodthorpe 2010).

That, indeed, is what metaphors do: they enable us to make sense of the world we live in – by understanding one reality through something else. Particularly those realities that are difficult to reach at because they are lacking a 'body', for instance 'God', 'death', and the stillborn child who leaves almost no traces behind, are being made sense off via the analogy of more tangible realities. Especially the sensuous 'world' of the body, objects, light, warmth and movement, is being called upon to grasp ephemere or abstract entities (Kövecses 2002). Therefore, death

2003 until 2009. This history is being published in Dutch under the title *Doodgeboren. Een mondelinge geschiedenis van rouw* (Amsterdam: De Bezige Bij 2012). (*Stillborn. An oral history of grief*). All names used in the text have been changed, in order to protect the participants' privacy.

becomes a 'transition' or 'ending'; we see in God a 'father' or 'judge', and the stillborn baby becomes present in the shape of a 'star' or 'gnome'.

Although hardly aware of this process, people cannot live without metaphors. Metaphors make order out of chaos (Fernandez 1972: 8). For instance, people can only relate to 'grief' by visualising it into something to think about and act upon. In contemporary society, grief generally is understand in terms of labour: inasfar as 'grief work' is what people do. The image is not without consequences, since people actually believe they can control grief through performing a set of tasks (Worden 1991); as long they we put enough effort into grief work, they will be rewarded by the end of the grieving process.

In other words, metaphors are far more than linguistic ornaments, they are ubiquitous (Lakoff and Johnson 1980: 453-457). They are not only present in speech, but also in embodied action. They form the meeting point of two landscapes: the landscape of inner thoughts, feelings and dreams, and the landscape of actions (see Garro en Mattingly 2000: 2-3). Thus, metaphors are situated both in people's heads and their movements. Moreoever, rather than being merely subjective or objective, they appear to be intersubjective: they are embodied within social interaction, and consequently they have a history.

In this chapter, to illustrate the performative work of hiding babies I discuss two approaches, told by a 57-year-old Flemish midwife called Ann who retired in 1999. She was highly aware of the differences between what she and some other narrators who participated in my research – an oral history of stillbirth – called a 'distant' and a more 'intimate' approach. Due to a reorganisation of midwifery services, she literally had to move from one approach to another, and her narrative evaluation of both ways of practicing – a dramatic contrast of opposites – is a more conscious one and portrays a highly pessimistic image of past practice'.

Ann's representation is not unique and through their repetition or emotional tone, most professional narratives highlighted the act of hiding as a key image of past practice. It is also worth noting that whereas midwives directly enagaged with the topic of stillbirth, gynaecologists tended to remain silent on the matter. Some midwives clearly felt guilty about their past roles and actions, whereas most doctors still used of a distant discourse.

Nevertheless, my aim is not to formulate a fixed typology of approaches differentiating midwives from gynaecologists or other professional groups. Rather, my intention is to explain the practice of hiding as a dynamic moment of meaning-making when a stillbirth occurs. Interestingly, the narrative representations of both past and present professional methods convey how the act of hiding deceased babies metaphorically brought forward concrete understandings of the space in which the stillbirth occurred, the baby's body, and the intangible idea of approprate grieving (Mitchell 2006).

In particular: as long as the baby was being hidden, the maternity ward became a 'conveyor belt', in that the baby became an 'object', and the existing grief model was litteraly being enacted in the act of 'letting go'. I discuss this in more detail next.

Conveyor Belt

As long as the stillborn baby was being hidden in hospital – in Flanders this was the case until the 1990s – death took place in a space resembling what I would call a 'conveyor belt'. Using exactly these terms, Ann described how she and her colleagues were supposed to act in a fast, cold and silent way.

The unwritten rule was clear: the stillborn baby had to be removed immediately. At least in her opinion, Ann had to treat both mothers and babies as 'serial products' with '800 deliveries a year' and in an economy of speed: 'we had to hurry, hurry, hurry'. But only if the baby appeared malformed or stillborn, it was removed abruptly and kept far away from the parents.

When something went wrong, 'it was sorted in an ice-cold way. I cannot stress enough how cold we were', said Ann. Showing emotions would have been a sign of unprofessionalism, according to one 87-year-old ex-midwife, who reported her 'mistake' of having shown emotions at the occasion of stillbirth: 'I once made the mistake of crying. At such moments you'd better not show any emotions. Not as a nurse or doctor, because then, you're saying you've made an error. You could be accused afterwards.' Crying could also be interpreted as an act of rebellion against God who was still largely being regarded as the major cause of stillbirth. I heard one woman convey how her own mother already one day after the stillbirth commanded her in 1963 'to stop crying, because it is a selfish act since in Heaven, being so close to the Lord's Light, the baby could not be more happy'. Thus Ann not only had to hide the baby, she was supposed to conceal her own emotions as well.

Ann described the ward as a silent place. Talking to parents about the stillbirth was not allowed as she told me: 'If you did, it would cause resentment and you'd be put on the carpet'. Ann still heard the head midwife, an older nun, expressing anger: 'What did you say to those people?' 'Everything was done in secrecy', she continued. 'Stirring as little emotions as possible. And keeping it quiet.' Equally, some parents would leave the hospital without being told that their stillborn baby had Down's syndrome.

It is remarkable how mostly negatively 'the nuns' are portrayed. Maybe it was held against them to be delegated the running of the maternity clinic without any real knowledge of motherhood. Furthermore, I would speculate that in a catholic country the depiction of imperious nuns might stem from childhood memories at school – of hierarchy, opposition and rebellion against religious authority in general.

When talking about these practices surrounding stillbirth, the midwife and many other professionals expressed emotional, uncomfortable or just bad feelings. It was a 'mentality' that Ann now found 'was breaking her down'. By referring to 'rules', 'circumstances', a 'mentality', 'habit' or 'approach' birth professionals were indicating a way of acting that belonged to everyday life.

Indeed, the practice of hiding was taken-for-granted as Ann told me: 'We had the feeling that we had to behave that way: not showing too much compassion, trying not to talk about it all the time, hushing it up.' The so-called fast, cold and silent sphere in which hiding occurred, can be understood as part of the everyday distant approach of hospital life. With hindsight, Ann found it 'awfully old-fashioned' or even 'medieval'. But Ann also reported that she 'didn't have any space to behave differently', thereby interpreting hiding as something situated within social and institutional constraints outside her individual will: 'I had troubles with it, but it was just like that, and you had to, you couldn't escape from it and do it differently, that wasn't possible.'

So, being a midwife in the 1970s was not only represented as 'stressful' but also frustrating. Ann 'wasn't given any freedom' by the gynaecologist who 'was a tyrant' and because 'the nuns' rules still prevailed even though they were no longer there. One midwife, practising from 1960 until 2002, called this everyday life in which the act of hiding should be situated, a 'system' that was governed by one authoritive and strict religious woman: 'You always had to take away the dead baby, and if the mother asked: 'can I see my baby?', it was not allowed. That was heartbreaking. After a while, I didn't care anymore. So the moment the sister would leave the building I showed the baby anyway. I think that was a good cause.' However, Ann did not rebel and now finds it 'bizarre' and 'unbelievable' that she and her colleagues kept doing things in that way. In the end however, she was able to escape from this prison-like image of the distant approach since 'later on, all that did change'. Having to move to another hospital in 1995 following a reorganisation, Ann and her colleagues were not only entering another ward but also 'a totally different approach to the situation': one of 'openness'. She represented this experience as a 'confrontation' entailing a 'complete turnover', one which asked for 'adaptation':

> I didn't see it change because we had only been confronted with it in the other hospital. The mother could help washing the little dead child, being dressed and held it in the room as long as they wanted to, and then it was brought to the basement again until they would ask 'can I have it again for a while?', which they always could, so they could take it closely with them. People could handle that little child, they could do what they wanted, watching it, making pictures, the little feet and hands were, they were inked, and then you had a souvenir.

Hiding babies no longer created a space resembling a conveyor-belt or transformed the ward into one that was more formal than it had been a moment ago. No longer feeling herself to be at the mercy of a rigid regime of taken-for-granted rules, Ann now had to adjust to a more intuitive way of practising in a ward atmosphere that was no longer 'fast, cold or silent'.

For her the performance of 'showing' the stillborn baby and the slow, warm and communicative practices revealed a new 'habitus' (Bourdieu 1990). It transformed the space into a place of 'openness', one resembling a personal and informal home in which actions appeared spontaneous: 'There was nothing to it, one knew how to behave on such occasions.' In contrast to the former approach, the latter was evaluated positively.

The 'dramatic' contrast between the two scenes which Ann and the other professionals narratively constructed during interviews is revealing (Garro and Mattingly 2000). In countering any accusation of being responsible or to blame for any pain caused to parents, in her representation of past experiences, sometimes in reported speech, Ann was identifying herself as an emotional, innocent and caring midwife. Leaving behind what she called the 'old-fashioned' distant approach, however, cannot soley be explained by changes in authority or power.

Ann referred to other contextual shifts, mostly in technology. It is true that the advent of ultrasound images during the 1970s, and more regularly in the 1980s, changed the professional confrontation with stillbirth. Able to detect non-viability at an early stage of pregnancy, birth professionals mostly did not have to cope with the shock of, more frequent, unanticipated stillbirth. The rather slow process of communication which involved giving parents their say on the decision about viewing their stillborn baby could begin before the actual delivery. Indeed, the specific practice of the hiding cannot be understood separately from these new conditions of possibility.

It is, nevertheless, important to note that the 'hiding' approach has been described as a 'belief' that it is the right thing to do, an ideological act far more than an effect of power relations or technological possibilities. As I will show, the distant hiding was, more or less consciously, believed to have had a salutary influence on parents.

Object

I argue that through the act of hiding stillborn babies, embodied subjects – in this case professionals, parents and babies – were both confirmed and located in certain positions and roles. Further, the body of the stillborn baby was the trigger for this distant practice of hiding transformed stillborn bodies which contrasts significantly with contemporary intimate practice. By taking a baby away from parents speedily and silently, midwives and gynaecologists found themselves transformed into more authoritative and professional bodies whose firm agency overode that of babies' parents. Ann interpreted the wooden, distant behaviour of the gynaecologists as a result of their feelings of awkwardness. She told me,

> If everything ended well, they were playing the big shot. But in sad situations, they didn't know what to do. They were experts, though, but as to contact with the people, they were very stiff.

An old and formerly reputatable Flemish professor in gynaecology maintained that he 'probably did what around and before' him was done, further confessing on behalf of his profession: 'we failed in our duties because it was so painful to go and explain in front of these people'.

By contrast, during the performance by professionals of hiding their babies parents were denied agency insofar as hiding could render them passive 'patients' not able to act autonomously. Discursive repertoirs such as 'they could (not)' or 'they were (not) allowed to' conveyed the extent to which in the distant approach to stillbirth, power and decision making were not shared with them. Parents were acted for, and, moreover, kept in ignorance: 'the less they knew, the better', said Ann.

I argue that the baby, was the most hybrid body in the ward, in that it was less a subject and more an object. The process of hiding moved him or her out of the symbolically troublesome space of liminality. Because its face was not seen by its parents, its body not touched and not given an official name, the baby was depersonalised. In this way, the stillborn baby could remain an abstract idea to the parents, rather than a concrete, tactile and physical being and person.

This objectification was also enshrined in law. In Belgium until 1999 local government offices were not allowed to write down the christian name of a stillborn baby. Hence the birth certificate mentioned a 'dead child of the (fe)male sex'. Furthermore, as it was also the practice in Belgium, the town hall registered the stillborn baby under the name of its mother thus connecting the baby to the woman's body as so-called reproductive failure. At the hospital, women were often placed in a general ward following stillbirth, not with other mothers of live babies and were thus, treated as sick women (Lovell 1983).

However, a more 'positive' interpretation of the practice following stillbirth is possible. Not being held, photographed or captured in any way, the baby could take on divine qualities. Being unapproachable and without image could make stillborn babies sacred. What I mean by this is that a stillborn child came from the invisible world of the womb and was God's creation, and staying in this invisible world, kept it free from earthly pollution. The stillborn baby embodied a reality which transcended men and women and was therefore considered dangerous. Hiding the baby was equal to laying it in the hands of Gods. Older nurses told me how a stillborn baby was often surrounded by plugs of cotton, resembling heavenly clouds.

In her seminal work *Purity and danger* (1966) the anthropologist Mary Douglas explains how realities and situations have to be ritually averted because they embody boundaries in themselves and challenge the symbolic ways of ordering the world. From this viewpoint, the stillborn child is such a reality: dying at the moment it entered the world of the living, the baby seemed to be neither alive nor dead, rather both alive and dead at the same time. This highlights in a most painful way how birth is not simply birth, and death no longer just death. Rather, stillbirth is a reminder of the fragility the meanings people have created, even those thought of as obvious. Further, stillbirth also highlights how fragile the boundaries are between life and death, and how suddenly the world – previously understood through clear categories – can turn into chaos (see Howarth 2001).

In the more recent intimate practice following stillbirth, birth professionals showed a new dimension to their authority: at stake now their self image of an empathetic carer, rather than an aloof curer. Professionals have become the actors, script authors and performance directors. Parents are asked to choose based on the information that professionals provide.

In this intimate approach, the act of showing the stillborn baby could alter the hybrid body in another way, with the baby's body transformed into a 'more human' one. And this is only the first step, for (depending on the parents' wishes) showing the baby could be followed by holding, clothing, cuddling, washing and photographing and through this performance parents become more like traditional parents.

However, hiding stillborn babies is sometimes still considered to be the best practice. For example, seriously disfigured babies would still be hidden to avoid traumatic memories. I argue that in a symbolic sense, on these occasions the practice of showing the baby would mean that its subjectivity could be threatened and its personhood endangered. While hiding confirmed the stillborn baby as object, in this specific example, the process of hiding highlights a performance of the oppposite. The intimate approach of showing the stillborn baby affirms the double or hybrid character of the baby's body including both physical and social aspects yet performing and prioritising the latter (see Hockey 2001).

Letting Go

Finally, past and present 'good practice' reflect corresponding approaches to the ideas of death and grief. Hiding the baby's body, moreover, created a space for specific images through which to experience both death and grief in a direct, tactile way. I suggest that the older stillbirth practice of hiding brought 'intimate death' into being whereas the intimate approach performs a 'distant death'.

The concepts of intimate and distant death (Bleyen 2005) together encompass a comprehensive notion of 'death' that illuminates some of the paradoxes. Distant death concerns that of an unknown and object-like being; a process outside of the self, in which one is not really touched or involved (Bleyen 2009). The narrative representations of past practices and experiences by birth professionals clearly suggest that it was this kind of death which was being performed through hiding stillborn babies.

Just as other death professionals (such as pathologists whose task is to dissect the body) depersonalise the corpse, hiding the baby also rendered it as an object, rather than a subject. For doctors, death at the hour of birth and the search for an explanation took place behind closed doors, or, drawing on Goffman's (1959) dramaturgical metaphor 'back stage' (unseen by the audience), with the baby subjected to autopsy and scrutiny. For birth professionals, whose task it is to 'produce' new life – (note the conveyor-belt metaphor used earlier) – death is a most disturbing reality. Ariès (1981) who argued that death was sequestered might have claimed that the hiding of the stillborn baby was in fact hiding death.

Indeed, the medical discourse is one in which life and death, the latter considered a technical challenge, are dichotomised. Or as one older paediatrician reported: 'One cannot let the child stay among the other living children. That is evident'. Parents were not only kept passively at a safe distance from the body of their child, the performance of hiding it also made sense of their future relationship with the child: spatially and symbolically securing a firm boundary between life and death as well as separating the living from the dead. The dead baby could not to be integrated into its parents' 'future social lives or life as a whole. In other words, as long as birth professionals were making the uniform decision to hide the stillborn infant, they were encouraging the grieving parents to let go of it. Hiding stillborn babies thus affirmed the then popular model in which 'grief was eventually resolved by detaching, letting go and moving on to new relationships' (Walter 1999: xiii). Furthermore, birth professionals – and many other social actors outside the hospital – would often avoid openly acknowledging parents' relationship with the baby and thus socially accept their loss. In this way, the unspoken or explicit order to let go is, exemplary of a 'disenfranchised grief' (Doka 2002). Indeed, according to some professionals, parents did not grieve in the first place. One gynaecologist argued that 'since the world view was still completely different, maybe, those mothers weren't given great support from the hospital because their urge wasn't that great.' Or as Ann explained the practice of hiding:

> It must have been the remains of earlier days when enormous amounts of children died at birth, and it wasn't seen yet as something abnormal. In order to console, people used to say that it was happening all the time. I don't know whether people, having so many children, used to experience as much as sorrow when one of them dropped out. I sometimes wonder, but one doesn't find answers.

According to Layne (2003), mothers are believed to grieve more intensely today than ever, as they fall into a difficult cultural gap between increased prenatal bonding and unrealistic expectations about pregnancy outcomes; a cultural taboo on the death of a baby due to western ideas of progress.

Accepting that to a great extent grief is socially and culturally constructed, does not necessarily mean that decades ago, mothers and fathers experienced less pain. Yes, because of the dominant discourse at that time, they grieved in a *different* way, and the pain articulated through other (religious instead of psychological) words and references but since the 1990s the practice of hiding and the model of letting go both have been challenged.

When Ann witnessed for the first time how a stillborn infant was shown and given to its parents, she was confronted with another kind of death in the ward: intimate death. In contrast to distant death, intimate death is the death of a subject intertwined with, in this case, parents' (and to a less extent also staff's) own life and personhood, in such a way that it was impossible to experience death at a distance. It implies a real, partial loss of the *self*. Therefore, it cuts into one's guts: it hurts, upsets and alters life for good (Bleyen 2005: 24-25, Malkinson 2001: 223).

In contrast to hiding, the act of showing destabilised the binary opposition or boundaries of 'life' and 'death'. The performance of intimate death clearly acknowledged what I call their hybridity. Although the baby was biologically dead it nevertheless retained an important social presence in the lives of the parents and other intimates. By dressing, cuddling, naming and so on, the stillborn baby could yet become a son or daughter. The baby was treated as if alive. I argue that the stillborn baby was being moved between its 'two bodies': its biological body which had died, and its social body either the son or daughter to be. Hence the body that more than merely an 'it', rather metaphorically it became a 'name', for instance 'Julie' or 'Peter' and by a series of practices it was given an imagined future and a social identity (see Hallam and Hockey 1999: 74).

In general, ward power and authority moved from the doctor and his or her professional expertise, which meant always hiding stillborn babies to that of parents' personal choice between showing or hiding. My data show that in Belgium the psychological discourse of expressing feelings became dominant over the medical one of silence as the only response to stillbirth. In short, the shift from hiding towards showing (or hiding if necessary) lays bare the shift towards a so-called 'post-modern' death (Walter 1996: 195).

Indeed, whereas medical professionals still show a prior interest in the cause of death, midwives tend to focus on the well-being of parents – especially that of the 'mother', referring to 'men' rather than 'fathers'. Men are seemingly not fully constructed as fathers, neither in past practices, nor in current narratives, since theire bodily connection to the child is less clear. This well-being is no longer situated in a grief model of letting go, but rather one of 'continuing bonds' (Valentine 2008). Revealing that his own sister had lost a baby three decades ago, a 74-year-old priest, who had worked in hospital since 1978, talked sensitively and openly about stillbirth. He clearly subscribed to the grief model of continuing bonds as he talked, gently addressing bereaved parents about the value of naming:

> If you would call it Mary, or no matter how, but you would be able to pronounce it with all your sorrow and carry it later on with you in your heart.

Final Comments

In the course of the last century, conceptions of death have changed radically. From a transition to a true existence in the light of the Lord, at least in formerly catholic contexts within western societies, is now the end of life. Funeral rites were not meant to contribute to the development of a personal image of a beloved one and the emotional care of the survivors, since as long as death was not an ending and people were not considered to live on in one's memory, funerary rites provided a safe and sound portal for the Christian's soul to enter heaven through set formulas, prayers and indulgences (Bleyen 2005). This altered face of death was also being enacted in the ward where occasionaly a mother gave birth to a dead child. When the stillborn child was taken away to another room, the baby would undergo a transition to a different and invisible world.

However, religious ideas were not all that lay behind the act of hiding babies. Rather, the shift towards showing babies happened in all kinds of context within recent European history, hence revealing broader cultural changes. For instance: the grown value of memory-making in general and the importance of the body in particular. The vulnerable boundary between life and death which the stillborn baby unravelled was not supposed to be experienced by parents. The stillborn baby was 'dangerous' because it brought a strange and threatening reality close that did not seem to fit the categories through which time and space and other dimensions were understood. As explained by Hallam, Hockey and Howarth (1999) like any other corpse, the dead baby revealed how limited our control is over the body, how fragile are our identities, and how uncivilised our body is in reality. By being born and simultaneously dying, the stillborn baby occupied the boundary between life and death and was particularly painful because it threatened the security of that boundary. Moving the baby's body to a confined place, symbolically lifted it over the boundary. In my interpretation, the act of carrying away the baby and keeping it somewhere else symbolically resealed the newly porous boundary between life and death (Bleyen 2012). Indeed, far from being merely physiological reactions to personal experiences, perceptions are arenas of social interaction (Howes 2003: xi; Bendix 2005). The radical experience of stillbirth thus coincided with a totally new sensory perception, not only of the baby's body itself and the physical space of the ward, but also of the abstract concepts of death and grief. Whereas in the past 'hiding' stillborn babies assured a bodily distance between parents and their child, contemporary 'showing' of the stillborn baby secures proximity.

So, when Alice, a 30-year old therapist, gave birth to her stillborn son in 2004, her first child, she wanted to have him close to her: 'the nurse told me how the gynaecologist had said: 'how much do I wish I could blow life into him.'

References

Ariès, P. 1981. *The Hour of Our Death.* New York: Alfred A. Knopf.

Bendix, R. 2005. Introduction: ear to ear, nose to nose, skin to skin. The senses in comparative ethnographic perspective. *Etnofoor*, 18(1), 3-14.

Bleyen, J. 2005. *De dood in Vlaanderen. Opvattingen en praktijken na 1950.* Leuven: Davidsfonds Uitgeverij.

Bleyen, J. 2009. Defining and conceptualising death, in *Encyclopedia of Death and the Human Experience*, edited by C. Bryant and D. Peck. Thousand Oaks: Sage.

Bleyen, J. 2012. *Doodgeboren.* Amsterdam: De Bezige Bij.

Bourdieu, P. 1990. *The Logic of Practice.* Cambridge: Polity Press.

Burke, P. 2005. Performing history: the importance of occasions. *Rethinking History*, 9(1), 35-52.

Cecil, R. 1996. *The Anthropology of Pregnancy Loss. Comparative Studies in Miscarriage, Stillbirth and Neonatal Death.* Oxford and Washington: Berg.

Doka, K.J. (ed.) 2002. *Disenfranchised Grief. New Directions, Challenges, and Strategies for Practice*. Champaign Illinois: Research Press.

Edvardsson, D., Rasmussen, B.H. and Riessman, C.K. 2003. Ward atmospheres of horror and healing: a comparative analysis of narrative. *Health: an interdisciplinary journal for the social study of health, illness and medicine*, 7(4), 377-396.

Fernandez, J.W. 1972. Persuasions and performances: of the beast in every body. And the metaphors of everyman. *Daedalus. Journal of American academy of arts and sciences, myth, symbol and culture*, 101(1), 39-60.

Garro, L.C. and Mattingly, C. 2000. Narrative as construct and construction, in *Narrative and the cultural construction of illness and healing*, edited by L.C. Garro and C. Mattingly. Berkeley and London: University of California Press, 1-49.

Goffman, E. 1959. *The Presentation of Self in Everyday Life*. New York: The Overlook Press.

Hallam, E., Hockey, J. and Howarth, G. 1999. *Beyond the Body. Death and Social Identity*. London and New York: Routledge.

Hockey, J. 2001. Body, Two Bodies Theory, in *Encyclopedia of death and dying*, edited by G. Howarth and O. Leaman. London: Routledge, 57-58.

Hockey, J., Komaromy, C. and Woodthorpe, K. (Eds). 2010. *The Matter of Death: Space, Place and Materiality*. Basingstoke: Palgrave Macmillan.

Howes, D. 2003. Introduction: Empire of the senses, in *Sensual relations. Engaging the senses in culture and social theory*, edited by D. Howes. Ann Arbor: The University of Michigan Press, 1-17.

Kellehear, A. 2007. *A Social History of Dying*. Cambridge, UK: Cambridge University Press.

Kövecses, Z. *Metaphor*. 2002. *A Practical Introduction*. Oxford: Oxford University Press.

Lakoff, G. and Johnson, M. 1980. *Metaphors We Live By*. Chicago: University of Chicago Press.

Layne, L.L. 2003. *Motherhood Lost. A feminist account of pregnancy loss in America*. New York and London: Routledge.

Lovell, A. 1983. Some questions of identity: late miscarriage, stillbirth and perinatal loss. *Social Science and Medicine*, 17, 756-757.

Malkinson, R. 2001. Grief, therapy, in *Encyclopedia of death and dying*, edited by G. Howarth and O. Leaman. London: Routledge, 223-225.

Mitchell, J.P. 2006. Performance, in *Handbook of material culture*, edited by C. Tilley, W. Keane, S. Kuechler-Fogden and M. Rowlands. London: Thousand Oaks, New Delhi: Sage, 384-401.

Polkinghorne, D. 1988. *Narrative Knowing and the Human Sciences*. New York: State University of NY Press.

Riessman, C.K. 2008. *Narrative Methods for the Human Sciences*. London: Sage.

Sontag, S. 1979. *Illness as Metaphor*. London: Random House.

Valentine, C. 2008. *Bereavement Narratives: Continuing Bonds in the 21st Century.* London: Routledge.

Walter, T. 1996. Facing death without tradition, in *Contemporary issues in the sociology of death, dying and disposal*, edited by G. Howarth and P.C. Jupp. London: Palgrave Macmillan, 193-204.

Walter, T. 1999. *On bereavement. The Culture of Grief.* Maidenhead and Philadelphia: Open University Press.

Worden, W. 1991. *Grief Counselling and Grief Therapy.* London and New York: Routledge.

Chapter 15
Managing Emotions at the Time of Stillbirth and Neonatal Death

Carol Komaromy

In this chapter I explore the emotional management of feelings in hospital settings following stillbirth and neonatal death. Each year in the UK nearly 6,500 babies are stillborn or die in the first 4 weeks of life. In 1990 the gestational age at which babies are classified as stillborn (rather than miscarried) was lowered from 28 to 24 weeks and meant that parents could register their baby's death and hold a funeral. Mothers and couples have been lobbying for recognition of the impact of stillbirth and neonatal death since the 1970s with some success and changes in practice have signified the need to handle such loss with sensitivity and compassion (Kohner 2001). For example, it is considered good practice for mothers and/or couples to spend time with their baby after birth and to keep mementoes such as photographs, hair, foot and handprints and for this to be a facilitative part of the grieving process (RCOG guidelines 1985 and see Bleyen, this volume, for a discussion of this change in practice in the Netherlands). This new response to stillbirth and neonatal death has impacted upon the way that midwives, obstetricians and gynaecological nurses and doctors practice and, in particular, the way that bereavement care is seen as a fundamental part of their role.

In this chapter, I explore what it means for midwives, women and couples to manage the emotions associated with perinatal death and draw exclusively on data from two interviews to illustrate some of the difficulties involved. One presents an example of loss from the perspective of a midwife and the other a grandmother. I draw on sociological theories of performativity and emotional labour to explain what might be happening at the level of interaction between professionals and parents. I also consider some implications for practice.

Being Professional at a Time of Loss

As a student midwife in the early 1990s working in the ante-natal clinic, an experienced midwife asked me to accompany her to break the news to a young woman aged about 17 years that her baby had died. This woman was attending the ante-natal booking clinic and had assumed that everything was fine but the ultra-sound scan revealed that her baby had died. She was with her mum and I remember clearly – as we sat in the room set aside for breaking bad news –

that it was raining hard and how the rain resembled tears on the windows. I also thought, 'she will remember every detail of this day for the rest of her life'. The senior midwife confirmed the news about the scan which the ultrasound technician had already disclosed and explained what would happen next. The young woman began to cry and her mother held her hand. Then the midwife said, 'You know, not all the seeds in the garden grow.' I was horrified. I had just completed my counselling training and here was someone teaching me how to communicate bad news in a way that I considered to be harmful.

The way that bad news is broken has improved to the extent that it takes account of individual diversity. Disclosure training is included in the curricula for doctors and nurses. It is also much more likely that midwives will be skilled in providing supportive responses to miscarriage, stillbirth and neonatal death. However, the reflection above illustrates my interest in the need for compassion as part of a professional role. It also illustrates the way that I made a judgement on the quality of the disclosure and my personal belief that the nature of how bad news is broken can add to or mitigate the harm. As a sociologist, concerned that research should impact on practice, I wonder if prescribed forms of managing grief following stillbirth and neonatal death might not provide the space for the expression, or lack of display, of a range of emotions. Regardless of what is expected of practitioner roles in terms of the demands around breaking bad news and offering support, midwives and nurses (and many other professional groups such as ultra sound technicians, obstetricians and gynaecologists) need to present a professional demeanour which involves the management of their *own* feelings. The 'permission' that has been given to women and couples to show their emotions after the death of their baby is afforded by the practitioners who care for them during and after the events of birth and death. This is promoted through protocols that have developed to better facilitate the grieving process – but these protocols do not mean that all emotions are acceptable and the experience of loss is assumed to be a painful and sad one. I argue that within the new orthodoxy of handling stillbirth and neonatal death, professionals and parents alike are expected to respond appropriately according to this orthodoxy. It is the way that this is managed that is central to this chapter.

Sociological theory is useful in explaining the construction of professional responses, not only by challenging the assumptions on which expectations about the management of feelings are based, but also in highlighting the dangers that are inherent in any prescribed forms of behaviour. For example, in Hochschild's (1983) seminal work on the airline industry, she argued that people employed to work in commercial companies needed to do more than the tasks required of them; they also needed to regulate their emotions according to the expectations of the organisation. She argued further that, as much as the service which airline staff delivered to passengers, also what was being sold was a 'professional demeanour' in the form of producing the right emotions that would make passengers feel good. At the time of her study, there was a clear division of labour with most of the crew (called stewardesses) comprising women doing 'women's work'.

The professions of nursing and midwifery, the practitioners most often involved in the care of women and couples following stillbirth and neonatal death, are populated almost entirely by women and it is part of their role to present a professional emotional demeanour as part of the service they provide. (See Mitchell and Smith (2003) on learning disability nursing, Smith and Gray (2000) on nursing and, McQueen (2004) on negative emotions.) Indeed, the reality is that the emotional responses of practitioners such as nurses and midwives are prescribed by the protocols of the institution and the professional discourses that prevail. Institutional norms have always framed professional behaviour in health care even though changes in protocols themselves might be influenced at the clinical, social and political level.

Critiques of Hochschild highlight the over-simplification of her theory of emotional labour. For example, James (1982) has offered a more nuanced interpretation that allows for the recognition of a greater degree of negotiation and individual diversity within the emotional expressions of professionals in caring roles. However, as a basis from which to challenge assumptions about responses to death, including those of practitioners, Hochschild's concept remains a useful tool.

The expectation of the needs of women and couples following stillbirth and neonatal death is that they will benefit from seeing and holding their baby and is part of a new orthodoxy of grief. Thus, while in the past, parents were expected to cope better by forgetting the experience of a stillbirth or neonatal death, expert knowledge based on new theoretical models of grief suggests that it is of benefit to parents' mental health to spend time with their dying and deceased baby (see Lewis, 1979 on the need to touch and hold deceased babies in order to facilitate mourning and Kubler-Ross, 1970 on facing the reality of death). This is in keeping with the normative expectation that people are more likely to recover from loss if they express their feelings and are encouraged to talk. Despite this, a study published by Hughes et al. in the Lancet in 2007, contested the benefit of holding a stillborn baby, arguing instead that contact is associated with worse outcomes. Hughes et al. (2007: 6) who found that seeing and holding babies produced more trauma and poor longer-term outcomes argue:

> Staff are also shocked and upset when there is a stillbirth. Inexperienced staff might feel at a loss to know what to say or do, and perhaps the protocol (of parents seeing and holding their dead infant) gives them reassurance that there is a 'right way' to manage the situation. This suggests that both practitioners and parents alike are dependent upon regulated guidelines on what is the best thing to do.

They argue also that it was their impression based on the study data, that mothers did not have any plan of how to manage the situation and simply went along with what was expected of them.

If it is the case that emotion rules framed by professional practice norms partly dictate how women and couples should feel after the death of their baby, offering support to women and families in a way that recognizes the authenticity of their feelings is challenging.

Professional and Service User Demeanour

In what follows I draw on data from two interviews to highlight what happened at the time of death from the perspective of a practitioner and service user. I use pseudonyms to protect their identity. In the first interview, a midwife (an ex-colleague) whom I call Rosemary talked to me about managing the care of a woman and her baby following a stillbirth. In the second, a grandmother (also an ex-colleague) talked to me about what happened when her grandson died minutes after birth. I examine the extent to which their responses were social performances in that they produced a response that was in keeping with the new orthodoxy.

Midwives Managing Emotions

Rosemary had been a midwife for 10 years at a large teaching hospital in the West Midlands, in the UK. She described to me '*her* first stillbirth' which had occurred two years previously. Because the baby had died in utero, the stillbirth was anticipated and labour was induced. This case was assigned to Rosemary at the handover from the early to late shift in the labour ward. It is worth mentioning that the handover is a public event, during which the care of particular labouring women is assigned by the senior person in charge for that shift to the care of specific midwives on duty. The allocation of labouring women is not a negotiation – although, as you will note, there seemed to be scope for Rosemary to refuse to care for someone as she explained to me:

> R: I must admit my heart sank. I could have refused, well sort of, there's a choice but its Hobson's choice really – you know? If I didn't do it then one of the other midwives that shift would have had to and I would have felt – not just bad – erm – I mean guilty – but erm – not up to the job. And part of the job of a midwife is to look after women in all situations not just normal labour but when things go wrong.

She described what it was like to care for the woman during the labour and her account reflected her personal feelings of difficulty and distress. In this chapter I focus on what transpired after the birth. She told me how she carried out her role in the most supportive and professional way that she could. It was later, when she left the room to wash and dress the baby and return her to her mother, that she 'allowed' herself to reflect on her own feelings in this private space as she describes here:

R: So I took the baby out and washed and dressed her and tried to make her look good. She did not look good – she was really purple – almost black – and she was stained with meconium. It wasn't easy. I talked to her all the time.

I: Can you say more about talking to her?

R: Mmmm. It's interesting that. It's mostly to help *me* – it's just really hard to handle a still and silent baby – everything in us as midwives trains us for watching them at birth really carefully – checking that everything is normal and being ready to react if it's not. And, I guess deep down, you can't believe it either – deep down I can't accept it's happened and the baby lying there so still and so silent is the proof – that in some way we have failed this woman. And nobody wants to face that. Talking – it's a bit about being kind to the little thing that didn't make it and it's also about being distracted from the truth.

The extracts highlight the ways in which Rosemary managed her own emotions in order to be able to cope and appear to be professional. She expressed the need to demonstrate how as a midwife she should be able to look after women even when things go wrong as a strong rationale for doing what she did not want to do. Further, in terms of the role of the midwife and what it includes, stillbirth can represent the failure to deliver live and healthy babies. But the role also demands that midwives must be present, indeed it is illegal in the UK knowingly to give birth without calling for a midwife or doctor (Marland and Rafferty 1997).

Rosemary raised the issue of silence. The delivery room in a maternity unit is often noisy with the cries of a baby at the end of labour heralding a successful live birth. The silence that accompanies an anticipated stillbirth is something that midwives remark upon. Whether anticipated or not, a baby who does not cry suggests that there is something wrong. By using talk to ease her own discomfort of the silent baby, Rosemary was telling me how she coped with something that she found emotionally difficult. During the preparation of the baby for return to its mother, Rosemary was aware that she needed to make the baby look 'presentable' and ready to be viewed and held by its mother. From her description of the colour of the baby, this was difficult to achieve. She told me how she wrapped the blanket loosely around and slightly over the baby's face to help conceal some of the discolouration.

The next account is from Margaret whose grandchild died shortly after birth and who talked about the experience of seeing and holding a stillborn baby.

Expressing Grief following Neonatal Death

I knew Margaret well and I'd had many conversations with her about this event. Margaret was keen for her story to be used as part of research and we agreed that I would I interview her just under one year after her grandson's death. Beyond the need to contribute to improving the care of people in her situation and to participate in my small study, she welcomed the opportunity to talk about her grandson's death. Further, Margaret called me a week later to tell me that she had found the interview therapeutic and I have wondered if this had provided a legitimate space for her own feelings – given that the entire focus was upon the grief of her daughter (and remains so).

Margaret recalled how late one evening she went to look after Mark – her first grandson – while her daughter Laura who was in labour and her partner, Bob, went into hospital. Early the next morning, Margaret received a phone call from Bob to tell her that Laura had given birth to a son (Jack) but that it was unlikely he would live. He had died before Margaret and Mark could get to the hospital. She left Mark with his father in the waiting area and went to comfort Laura. Jack had died just minutes after birth, although the attempt to resuscitate him had been prolonged. The following extract describes Margaret's first meeting with Jack:

> ... And he was just like a real baby and that was what was so shocking. I thought I was going to see a dead baby and it was a real baby. It was just a sleeping baby. And that was sort of unreal – my kind of enduring image is of her holding this baby and looking at him and he was wrapped up nicely and he looked – you know – a bit bluish/purplish, but not anything that you wouldn't expect of a newborn baby. And she had actually been sitting and holding him for two hours or so and I sat down and she said, 'Do you want to hold him?' And I almost – you know – couldn't – but then it was all so easy 'cos there was no way in which he was different from a wholesome baby. And actually, when I did hold him he was still warm and there was not anything different. And it was like – what does a dead baby look like? What is a dead baby? What is this?

This extract shows how Jack was given life status to afford comfort – he was warm, he looked like a 'wholesome' 'real' baby, and he was cuddled. While Laura and Margaret knew that Jack was dead, it was 'as if' he was still alive. While Jack was medically/biologically dead, he was kept alive socially within this liminal space which was sanctioned by the midwives as a time and space for farewells. It was within the relationship between mother (grandmother) and daughter (mother) that an identity for Jack was negotiated. They could get to know him through this potential for being 'real'. It is difficult to imagine how this could have been achieved if they had not been given access to Jack's body.

After a while a midwife came into the room and offered to take photographs. The use of photography as tangible proof of the existence of a baby is common practice in UK hospitals. Post-mortem photographs of babies are encouraged and most wards have good quality photographic equipment for such occasions (for a discussion on post-mortem photography see Hilliker 2006). The midwife took several photos and during the interview Margaret showed them to me. The extract that follows highlights the lack of protocol for responding to this practice and the ambiguity it produced:

> … There is this one of me with this dead baby in my arms looking at Laura and we just look like this little happy family group and when the midwife showed it to me, I said to her, 'put that away, just put that away, don't show it to her!' It was just so awful, I found it so shocking to see this and I was sort of looking at Laura and we just, really, – there we are with a new baby – you know? – And the experience wasn't – it certainly wasn't unpleasant or frightening, but it wasn't real somehow. But there was this immense sense of just awfulness as well – and sadness – so there wasn't any joy in this little thing, but it was quite comforting at the same time. It was a strange mixture of feelings, of not really engaging with the idea of a dead baby but somehow being comforted by him.

Margaret expressed feelings of ambiguity and embarrassment about the photograph and its inappropriateness. Despite the opportunity for Laura and Margaret to hold and handle Jack and the opportunity to say goodbye in this liminal space between birth and death Douglas (1984) argues that the boundary between life and death is both powerful and dangerous and needs to be managed. Events at the boundaries, here the boundary is between life and death, serve as useful reminders that people create rituals which are likely to be used to 'cope' with perceived dangers. I would argue that Margaret and Laura's feelings of ambiguity arose from not knowing how to behave, drawing on the experience of a photograph as a way of capturing a happy event, without being told what to do. Elias (1994) explains embarrassment as a social event in which an individual experiences the breaching of social prohibitions. The data illustrated that there was a degree of emotional management required of both Margaret and Rosemary in this situation. While they did not tell me that the experience of preparing the deceased baby and handing him or her to the parents and seeing and holding the baby was harmful, what emerged from the accounts was a concern about doing the right thing – for Rosemary this meant making the baby presentable so that its mother could experience the reality of the death and say goodbye and for Margaret it meant helping her daughter to cope by following the recommended procedure in being with Jack.

The Performance of Emotional Labour

I have argued elsewhere (Komaromy 2005), that the concept of emotional labour suggests that there is an authentic set of feelings which are being managed in as far as they are either being suppressed or produced. The lack of knowledge about how to respond in extraordinary situations suggests that the participants did not seem able to rely on their feelings and were more concerned with getting it right. I argue that as Elias (1994) claims, social scripts on how to behave are more powerful than authentic emotions. Indeed in certain situations, emotions have to be overcome in order to behave in the socially condoned way, recognising that this is subject to shifts over time. Beyond this, I argue the existence of 'authentic' emotion is contested.

Here Goffman's ideas about performativity (1959) are useful in helping to explain performance at a time of crisis and when the stakes are high such as the time of the collision between life and death. For example, the performance around the life-death boundary serves several purposes, not least to present an appropriate response that sustains the social (including institutional) requirements associated with death. Indeed for Goffman there was *only* the social self and even off-stage performances were social ones. However, the collision that takes place when death replaces life makes this separation between the authentic and the performing self difficult, if not impossible. It would seem that there is little or no script to respond to death when there was only one for life. Layne (1997) argues that the silence around pregnancy loss arises from the cultural denial of the possibility of anything other than a positive outcome during the ante-natal period. However, as the first extract from Rosemary highlights, the guidance that is given to midwives, who are the professional group most likely to manage this schism, includes preparation for coping with the silence that accompanies such events. Flint (1986) has written about the silence that usually accompanies a stillbirth and advocates ways of talking to the parents and baby during delivery as part of a midwives' role. She describes how the silence is often one of the most striking features of a labour room during the labour and an anticipated stillbirth. At times, she advises, midwives need to support women's achievement in labour in an equally positive way, regardless of the outcome, and also to give them permission to welcome their baby by offering an account of its progress and what it looks like at birth.

On an individual and personal level, the feelings produced by the loss of a baby at whatever age and stage are likely to be affected by any number of factors. Beyond this and at a cultural and social level, there are broader issues that explain why the event might be so problematic (Douglas 1984). While it is the case that parents in this situation of loss and terrible ambiguity will be in need of support and guidance, a prescribed expectation of how to respond would not allow for more authentic expressions of feelings to be expressed. For example, it is possible that a pregnant woman might feel relief or ambiguity at the loss of her baby and not able to show this when everyone is anticipating that she will be very upset. Further, some mothers might feel no need at all to see and hold their baby but feel constrained in expressing that lack of need. However practitioners', mothers' and couples' responses, are expressed, they are framed by expectations which are derived from institutional norms and script the way that all of them manage the right impression (Goffman 1959). Further, the role of emotional labour (Hochschild 1983) suggests that in health care at least, both service practitioners and bereaved family members are expected to manage emotions as part of that role. For example, it is clear from Rosemary's account that she was expected to behave in a professional manner which involved managing her emotions in ways that did not harm those in her care; however that harm was interpreted according to medical knowledge and the new orthodoxy of grief. Part of this orthodoxy involves an expectation that parents will want to hold their dead baby (Hughes et al. 2007). While parents are central to any care that is given, the need to protect their mental health and wellbeing scripts how the practitioners in this situation will behave and manage emotions. It could be argued that within this is room for an expression of diverse emotions. However, while parents are given access to the body of their deceased baby and encouraged to handle him or her, they are not guided in how to respond if they do not experience the grief reaction that is expected of them and there is some pressure to follow the new orthodoxy. Margaret said:

> I wasn't sure how long we were expected to stay with Jack and I have to admit to feeling it had been too long. I mean, I think we'd both had enough but we'd been told to have him for as long as we liked. Yet, it didn't seem right to say we'd had enough, and I could tell that Laura didn't want to hold him anymore. I was so relieved when the midwife came and offered to take him away.

Conversely, if mothers and couples want to spend much more time with their baby, the access that is given to parents to do so is likely to be limited by the number of requests for the baby to be brought to them and the length of time it seems reasonable to be with their baby. These points are based on my own professional practice in a neonatal unit where parents were concerned to do what was right and often asked for clarification.

The Implications of this for Practice

In conclusion, presenting the dead baby to women and couples immediately after the birth, as if he or she is living – as was the case in both of the interviews presented here – and the requirement for women and couples to cuddle him or her – as if it is a universal and intrinsic need for all parents, might present a relatively unproblematic shift in practice. Indeed, it is arguably better to offer the possibility than lose the chance, but I argue that cuddling a dressed and wrapped baby emphasizes how the actions of the midwives might script the performance. For example, the reality is that dead babies do not need to be dressed, cuddled and kept warm – their need is an assumed one by practitioners on behalf of bereaved women and couples. In other words, women are expected to treat their baby in the way that they might treat a new-born *living* baby. This presentation of the dead body as living (Howarth 1996) requires them to respond in a particular way. The important point here is that bereaved parents are encouraged to go along with a prescription of their own needs – regardless of how they might experience the events of stillbirth and neonatal death. The theory of performativity (Goffman 1959) would explain this by the way that threaded throughout this is the assumption that bereaved people will play their part in a response to death in an attempt to pull off a convincing performance of grief. Arguably though, the space that is set aside for facing death needs to be negotiated at an individual level, where the uniqueness of each event can be better appreciated and a one-size-fits-all approach challenged (also see Graham et al., this volume).

The theories of Goffman (1959) challenge the notion that anything is asocial and therefore the idea that there is an authentic self with authentic feelings is contested. Goffman was less interested in psychodynamic explanations of actions than the idea that all social beings have social connections to each other and are concerned with the impression that they make. While this does not fully explain the potential range and diversity of feelings at the time of stillbirth and neonatal death it highlights how institutional or theoretical norms that are imposed on reactions to death play a significant part in the performance of everyone involved in this type of death. While my argument is that the lack of clear scripts can leave parents floundering in terms of what to do at a very difficult time, I am also suggesting that it might be worse to offer them an inappropriate protocol on how to behave. I would argue that while protocols play a significant part in the care of bereaved women and couples, what people need most is a direct engagement which allows for an exploration of the best way to respond. Perhaps, as Layne (1997) argues, this cannot be left until it is too late to find out but needs to be anticipated and considered early on in the pregnancy, after all one has to know what to do the moment it happens.

References

Douglas, M. 1984. *Purity and Danger: An analysis of the concepts of pollution and taboo*. London: Kegan Paul.

Elias, N. 1994. *The Civilising Process: The history of manners*. Oxford: Blackwell.

Flint, C. 1986. *Sensitive Midwifery*. London: Heinemann Medical Books.

Goffman, E. 1959. *The Presentation of Self in Everyday Life*. London: Penguin Books.

Hilliker, L. 2006. Letting go while holding on: post-mortem photography as an aid in the grieving process. *Illness, Crisis & Loss*, 14(3), 245-269.

Hochschild, A. 1983. *The Managed Heart: The commercialisation of human feeling*. Berkeley, CA: University of California Press.

Howarth, G. 1996. *Last Rights: The work of the modern funeral director*. Amityville, New York: Baywood Publication Company.

Hughes, P., Turton, P., Hopper, E. and Evans, C.D.H. 2007. Assessment of guidelines for good practice in psychosocial care of mothers after stillbirth: a cohort study, *The Lancet* [Online] 360(9327), 114-118. Available at: doi:10.1016/S0140-6736(02)09410-2 [accessed14 December 2011].

James, N. 1982. Care= organisation + physical labour + emotional labour. *Sociology of Health and Illness*, 14(5), 488-509.

Kohner, N. 2001. *When a Baby Dies: the experience of late miscarriage, stillbirth and neonatal death*. London: Routledge.

Komaromy, C. 2005. The production of death and dying in care homes for older people: an ethnographic account. Unpublished thesis. Milton Keynes: The Open University.

Kubler-Ross, E. 1970. *On Death and Dying*. New York: Macmillan.

Layne, L.L. 1997. Breaking the silence: an agenda for a feminist discourse of pregnancy loss. *Feminist Studies*, 23(2), *Feminists and Fetuses* (Summer 1997), 289-315.

Lewis, E. 1979. Mourning by the family after a stillbirth or neonatal death. *Archives of Disease in Childhood*, 54(11), 303-306.

Marland, H. and Rafferty, A.M. 1997. *Midwives, Society and Childbirth: Debates and controversies in the modern period.* London: Routledge.

McQueen, A.C. 2004. Emotional intelligence in nursing work. *Journal of Advanced Nursing*, 47(1), 101-108.

Mitchell, D. and Smith, P. 2003. Learning from the past: emotional labour and learning disability nursing. *Journal of Learning Disabilities*, 7(2), 109-117.

Smith, P. and Gray, D. 2000. The emotional labour of nursing: how student and qualified nurses learn to care, Unpublished PhD thesis. South bank University: London.

RCOG (Royal College of Obstetricians and Gynaecologists). 1985. Report of the RCOG working party on the management of perinatal deaths. London: Chameleon Press, 1985.

Chapter 16

Experiences of Reproductive Loss: The Importance of Professional Discretion in Caring for a Patient Group with Diverse Views

Ruth Graham, Nick Embleton, Allison Farnworth, Kathy Mason, Judith Rankin and Stephen Robson

The kinds of healthcare available to parents who experience reproductive loss in the UK are varied. Partly, this results from experiences that can fall within the umbrella term of reproductive loss and which cut across the remit of several specialist providers of health care. Primarily these specialties are obstetrics, foetal medicine, gynaecology and neonatology, but may include others such as paediatrics and palliative care. In this chapter, the findings from our research on three different forms of reproductive loss (termination of pregnancy for foetal anomaly (TOPFA), withdrawal of life sustaining intervention in neonates, and miscarriage) are sampled heuristically to provide a cross-study insight into the way that diversity is interwoven into accounts of reproductive loss.[1] First, we map out some of the ways in which diversity of experience can be influenced by the organisation of formal health care experiences of conducting research in these three distinct areas of reproductive loss. Then, we use the case study of feticide prior to TOPFA to draw out in more detail some elements of diversity in experience within a particular area of healthcare. These two aspects of diversity highlight the importance of acknowledging the existence of different views (as a parent or as a professional) on the care pathways available for responding to reproductive loss. Acknowledging and responding to different views is crucial if good quality clinical care is to be provided. These aspects of diversity also emphasise the need for a level of professional discretion in clinical practice that allows clinicians to respond appropriately to such different views.

1 We would like to thank Helen Statham (Centre for Family Research, University of Cambridge, UK) for her contribution to the research projects that this chapter draws upon, and for her insightful comments on an earlier version of the chapter.

Understandings of Reproductive Loss

Some particular types of reproductive loss have been the subject of sociological or social science investigation. For example, termination of pregnancy (or induced abortion) has been a topic of interest to sociologists from an experiential point of view (such as Harden and Ogden's (1999) study of young women's experiences) as well as a useful case study to consider broader forms of social structure (for example, Ellie Lee's (2003) analysis of abortion and medicalisation in the US and the UK). In contrast, the concept of reproductive loss is a more recent one within sociology. The use of the concept became more formally acknowledged in a series of three articles published by an academic collaboration that incorporated a strong sociological component. In the first of these articles, Sarah Earle and her colleagues (Earle et al. 2007: 28) set out a list of forms of reproductive loss. Taking this list as a starting point, it is possible to sub-categorise the content in a way that highlights the multiple facets that contribute to understandings of reproductive loss in its different forms. In Table 16.1, some of these potential aspects are highlighted in a subdivision of the list provided by Earle et al. (2007):

Table 16.1 Forms of reproductive loss

Type of reproductive loss by medically defined term	Specific forms of loss associated with medically defined term
Category 1	
Infertility	Loss of reproductive identity + Loss of imagined child
Unsuccessful assisted conception	
Repeated early miscarriage	
Category 2	
Early/late miscarriage	Loss of imagined, healthy child + Loss of parent status
Stillbirth	
Neonatal death	
Infant death	
Termination of pregnancy for medical reasons	
Category 3	
Termination of pregnancy for non-medical reasons	Loss of pregnancy + Possibly loss of imagined child

Source: Adapted from a list taken from Earle et al. 2007: 28.

These categorisations are informed by our research experiences across several projects, and should be seen as exploratory, rather than definitive. We have found these categorisations useful in highlighting the similarities across our research into these three types of reproductive loss:

- *Category 1* includes situations where people have a desire to become parents but where this has not been possible without some form of medical intervention. In this sense, such experiences encompass the loss of (or an undermined sense of) successful reproductive identity, alongside the loss of an imagined child/family.
- *Category 2* includes forms of reproductive loss where the foetus is usually conceptualised as a baby (see for example Blizzard's (2007) discussion about the use of the term foetus/baby), and is defined as a 'wanted baby' (this is not limited to 'planned' pregnancies, but also encompasses those that have *become* a wanted pregnancy when the loss event took place). These types of reproductive loss often involve the loss of an established parent status, alongside the loss of the anticipated future healthy child.
- *Category 3* includes just one phenomenon; termination of pregnancy for non-medical reasons. The distinction made between termination of pregnancy for medical and non-medical reasons is important because it highlights the particular challenge of using the term 'wanted baby' as if it were simply an either/or issue. Termination of pregnancy for reasons other than foetal anomaly should not be automatically assumed to be of unwanted pregnancies.

In this chapter, we focus on examples from reproductive loss within category two; but while the examples drawn on also cut across several types of reproductive loss, they nevertheless represent just one section of a broader spectrum of experiences.

Researching Reproductive Loss

There are four research projects that we reflect on here. Three of these projects were qualitative, in-depth interview studies: parent and staff reactions to feticide prior to termination of pregnancy for foetal anomaly (Robson and Rankin 2003-6); parent and health professional experiences of treatment withdrawal from sick neonates (Robson, Embleton, Graham and Rankin 2006-9); and managing the expectation gap in healthcare following a miscarriage (Robson, Farnworth and Graham 2007). The fourth project was a survey-based study: providing feticide prior to termination of pregnancy for foetal anomaly: a survey of UK foetal medicine sub-specialists, (Graham, Robson, Rankin and Statham 2006-8) (see Table 16.2). Each project involved exploring understandings of a particular type of reproductive loss, but the issue of reproductive loss as a social problem was central to each project. In each of the four projects, attempts were made to

Table 16.2 Research projects

Study title	Study design	Number of participants	Response rates
STUDY A			
Parent and staff reactions to feticide prior to termination of pregnancy for foetal anomaly	Qualitative Semi-structured Interview study	14 Parents from 8 cases 23 health professionals	15-18% (parents) 88% (consultants) 33% (other medical) 70% (midwives)
Robson, S. and Rankin, J. 2003-6. *Parent and Staff Reactions to Feticide Prior to Termination of Pregnancy for Foetal Anomaly*. Funded by the Newcastle Healthcare Charity.			
STUDY B			
Parent and health professional experiences of treatment withdrawal from sick neonates	Qualitative Semi-structured Interview study	17 parents from 11 cases 25 health professionals	20% (parents) 78% (consultants) 63% (other medical) 50% (nurses)
Robson, S., Embleton, N., Graham, R. and Rankin, J. 2006-9. *Parent and Health Professional Experiences of Treatment Withdrawal from Sick Neonates*. Funded by Tiny Lives (UK Charity).			
STUDY C			
Managing the expectation gap in healthcare following a miscarriage	Qualitative Semi-structured Interview study	14 individuals from 9 cases 7 health professionals	60% (patients) n/a (consultants) 13% (other medical) 66% (nurses)
Robson, S., Graham, R., Farnworth, A. 2007. *Managing the Expectation Gap in Healthcare Following a Miscarriage*. Unfunded pilot study at Newcastle University.			
STUDY D			
Providing feticide prior to termination of pregnancy for foetal anomaly: a survey of UK foetal medicine sub-specialists	Self-completion Survey study	62 individuals from 21 separate FM units	76%
Graham, R., Robson, S., Rankin, J. and Statham, H. 2006-8. *Providing Feticide Prior to Termination of Pregnancy for Foetal Anomaly: a survey of UK foetal medicine sub-specialists*. Funded by the Newcastle University HASS Faculty Futures Programme.			

incorporate an element of post-structuralism thought into the analytic framework, to promote a 'reading' (Young 1990) of the data for instances of disputed meanings of what was considered problematic about reproductive loss. Therefore, we are able to draw on our involvement in this collection of projects to reflect on ways in which reproductive loss can be constructed as a legitimate social problem and a legitimate focus of social research.

Drawing on a broadly social constructionist perspective, Rubington and Weinberg's (1989: 4) introduction to social problems identified four key aspects of how such problems are evaluated: (i) the perceived reality of the situation; (ii) whether the identified issue is incompatible with core values; (iii) the number and significance of the individuals who find the situation problematic, and; (iv) whether action can be usefully taken. When considering reproductive loss, all four elements are relevant. Establishing whether a loss has taken place can be more challenging in certain circumstances (e.g. some forms of early miscarriage) but there is a growing sense that all three forms of loss discussed here have gained some degree of legitimacy as a 'real' issue at odds with broader social values. The state-funded health service in the UK provides services for such situations, and there are also voluntary organisations to support bereaved parents (for example, the Antenatal Results and Choices organisation (ARC), the Stillbirth and Neonatal Death charity (Sands) and the special care baby charity BLISS). The activities of these organisations demonstrate a belief that effective actions can be taken to support those who have experienced reproductive loss. For our purposes, it is the third criterion of the number and significance of the individuals who find the situation problematic which is of particular interest. This core community is probably best conceptualised as the parents of the lost foetus/baby and the staff who provide their care during or after the loss experience (whilst recognising that a wider social circle, including immediate family, can also be profoundly affected). This community will be larger for the more common types of reproductive loss, but a larger affected one does not necessarily translate into a more established status as a social problem. While it is not the purpose of this chapter to attempt to provide precise estimates of the number of reproductive losses that take place each year, it is possible to provide a thumbnail sketch of how the phenomena of feticide, neonatal death and miscarriage differ in frequency.

Of the three forms of loss discussed here, reproductive loss involving feticide prior to TOPFA is – numerically – the least common. In this context, feticide is a medical procedure that is used in late termination of pregnancy, to ensure that the foetus is not born alive, that is, showing signs of life (see Graham et al. 2009). The figures publicly available for feticide and late TOPFA are not easy to interpret, partly due to reporting restrictions on the basis of confidentiality and because of the very small numbers involved as the gestation of the pregnancy increases toward the threshold of viability. However, at the most, feticide represents approximately half to one per cent of total annual termination of pregnancy, and TOPFA approximately one per cent of total annual termination of pregnancy (DH 2003-11). Given that the overall termination of pregnancies in England and Wales has not yet exceeded 200,000, it seems reasonable to estimate that at the most, feticide prior to TOPFA is unlikely to involve the care of more than 1,500–2,000 patients per year, and can be considered a relatively rare experience. Drawing on England and Wales figures from national data on births, perinatal and infant mortality (CMACE 2011), it is possible to provide some approximate estimates for neonatal death. Estimating the number of miscarriages per year is more complex since no formal reporting procedure exists, but epidemiological studies can be used to provide a rough estimate.

Miscarriage, as a form of reproductive loss, is far more common. Estimates of the number of miscarriage are not definitive, but range between 20-30 per cent of conceptions (Wilcox et al. 1988, Simmons et al. 2006, Sur et al. 2009). If we were to consider the current level of miscarriage to be approximately 25 per cent of the rate of reported conception (ignoring the number of affected, but unreported, pregnancies), the estimate of miscarriages per year would be in excess of 200,000. Miscarriage is not an 'everyday' experience for all women, but it is certainly more commonly experienced than feticide prior to TOPFA.

Neonatal death (in particular, when preceded by active decisions to withdraw life sustaining support), appears to occur somewhere between these two positions, but nearer the less common end of the spectrum. Not all neonatal deaths involve the withdrawal of life-sustaining support, as some babies may not experience this particular type of care pathway (for example, if the baby dies too quickly for life sustaining support to be established). However, with this consideration in mind, and using the overall number of neonatal deaths reported in 2009, in the first 28 days of life the total figure is reported as 2511 (CMACE 2011). This figure does not include all deaths following withdrawal of life-sustaining support on a neonatal intensive care unit, as some babies die after 28 days; but it provides some indication of the lower threshold. These estimates suggest that reproductive loss in the neonatal period is slightly more common than reproductive loss involving feticide, but far less widely experienced than miscarriage.

Comparing estimates of the relative frequency of the different types of reproductive loss is important because it highlights the possible impact of loss on the organisation of formal health care and on issues of resource allocation. The most obvious aspect of this organisation is explored usefully by thinking about the impact of provision fragmentation. For neonatal death, and TOPFA, the healthcare provision is concentrated in, and developed by clinicians within one particular specialty – neonatal intensive care, and foetal medicine respectively. While other specialty groups may contribute, the care pathway has a well-established location within the current structural organisation of healthcare. In contrast, the care of those experiencing a miscarriage has developed in the UK in a much more patchy manner, despite the development of national guidelines (Hinshaw, Fayyad and Munjuluri 2006, Association of Early Pregnancy Units (AEPU) 2007); this type of reproductive loss has no obvious specialty to call home within the current National Health Service (NHS) structures, and can be housed in a range of organisational locations (for example see Cameron et al. 2007). Even limiting consideration to secondary care, people experiencing miscarriage might be cared for within a dedicated early pregnancy unit, a maternity or a gynaecology ward. Our own research in the areas of miscarriage, termination of pregnancy and neonatal death suggests that for most participants, the care provided was experienced as sensitive and helpful, and of a good standard. However, for the form of reproductive loss that is much more common (hospital managed) miscarriage, both patients and staff seemed overall less satisfied with the care provided. We cannot present definitive evidence of an association between: (1) the position within the hierarchy of the structural organisation of formal healthcare; (2) unit resource per reproductive loss event; and (3) levels of satisfaction with care provided for different types of reproductive loss; but we think this observation is interesting enough to warrant further exploration in future research. Certainly, the ways in which the formal organisation of health care might influence how professionals respond to reproductive loss are made more obvious. This diversity of location within the structural organisation of health care provision provides the backdrop against which other forms of diversity must be considered.

Diversity in Experiences of Reproductive Loss

In the investigation of health related phenomena, interpretative or qualitative social research is becoming more accepted by those researching and evaluating clinical practice and service provision (for example, see the dedicated chapters on this in Greenhalgh (2006) and Ajetunmobi (2002)). However, as Silverman (2006) notes, the focus of interpretative analysis often emphasises the possibility of multiple interpretations, rather than providing one definitive 'truth' to guide practice. This pluralism can be difficult to incorporate into the more dominant quantitative epistemological framework that governs medical research more generally. In terms of the research we have conducted on reproductive loss, this tension is played out in the acknowledgement and accommodation of diversity of views between staff and patients, and within these participant groups. Dealing with loss can be demanding and difficult work (Bolton 2005, Chiappetta-Swanson 2005) and the emotional work associated with this should not be underestimated (Hunter 2005). It is understandably tempting for clinical practitioners to seek out *the* best way to respond at the expense of developing knowledge to support a package of diverse responses. The tension between the notion of singular 'best' practice and more pluralistic 'good' practice is evident in attempts to develop guidelines on issues relating to reproductive loss. A recent debate surrounding guidance on offering parents the opportunity to see and hold their baby after death provides an example of this (see a health professional discussion site noting changes to the NICE guidance following discussion with SANDS representatives (MIDIRS 2010)). Similar to the views expressed by Judith Schott and Alix Henley (Schott and Henley 2008, Henley and Schott 2009), our research experiences and findings support the more pluralistic route to improving healthcare, giving parents meaningful choices wherever possible. Our findings have highlighted consistently the diversity of views on the part of both parents and staff, and the importance of sufficient discretion to allow parents and staff to co-produce a care pathway that is able to tolerate individual preferences within reasonable boundaries. In the remainder of this chapter, we present a number of examples that demonstrate such diverse experiences.

Example One: Experiences of Parent Status

This example is taken from the qualitative study of experiences of feticide prior to TOPFA (Table 2, Study A). The study included interviews with women and couples who had undergone a TOPFA. Some of the participants had been offered feticide, and some had not because they were not quite at the gestational threshold that triggers a routine offer of feticide as part of the termination process (21weeks+6days, RCOG 1996 and 2001). These two excerpts are taken from women who fell just below that threshold and therefore were not offered feticide:

> Well from the day we just discovered I was pregnant and decided to keep the baby, it became part of the family after that. [...] even though she hasn't come home, it's affecting all of us and our families (Feticide Study, Parent 4A&B, Mother).

> I don't feel like a parent. I think, had we left [the termination] any longer [...] one of the big things was that we didn't want to see the baby and we didn't want to know whether it was a boy or a girl. [...] I feel I've lost a pregnancy more than I feel like I've lost a baby (Feticide Study, Parent 23A, Mother).

These excerpts demonstrate that even within a small sample of eight cases, there was evidence of important diversity in how participants conceptualised themselves in terms of whether the foetus was a baby, or a 'pregnancy' with more or less emphasis on notions of parent and family identity. While the position represented by participant 4A was more typical within our small sample, participant 23A was not unique within the dataset. In another case in the same study, a participant described attempting to use the word 'foetus' rather than 'baby' as a deliberate strategy to protect themselves from the distress of what was happening. The potential for accommodating such diversity is limited by several factors including language; indeed, it is difficult to think of a usable concept that can encompass those individuals who experienced reproductive loss as parents, and those who experience it in ways that are less reliant on embracing an established parent identity.

Example Two: Conceptualisations of a 'Good Death' related to Termination of Pregnancy

This example is also taken from the qualitative study of experiences of feticide (Table 16.2, Study A), but the two excerpts included here are used to demonstrate diversity in how parents conceptualise a feticide procedure in the context of the 'good death' (Walter 2003) they wanted for the baby involved in a TOPFA:

> … if there was any sort of signs of life or any sort of fluttering I just wanted to hold [the baby] and just let her slip away (Parents 12 A&B, Mother, declined feticide).

> … it's kinder for the baby not to have to go through anything, the thought of giving birth to a baby prematurely having been you know, induced with lots of prostaglandins and everything and it has to go through birth and then it lives for a few hours, that doesn't make sense you know … if you're doing it for reasons of like reducing cruelty then that's pretty cruel (Parents 39 A&B, mother, accepted feticide).

The accounts of grief provided by parents in this study were similar regardless of whether or not feticide was offered, or accepted/declined. However, one of the few differences identified in the analysis related to the reasons parents gave for why feticide had been either accepted or declined. This difference related to understandings of what constituted suffering on behalf of the foetus/baby. Ultimately, the contrasting interpretations of what constitutes a 'good death' for the foetus/baby here highlight the subjective nature of understandings of suffering, and the difficulty of attempting to evaluate on philosophical grounds a singular notion of 'best' practice when multiple adequate care pathways exist.

Example Three: Using Discretion in the Provision of Termination of Pregnancy for Foetal Anomaly

This example is taken from a study of the views of consultants, who provide feticide prior to TOPFA (Table 16.2, Study D). The provision of late TOPFA is a complex issue in social and legal terms, and information that contextualises these issues can be found in Statham et al. (2006). In this example, we focus on a specific professional guideline that exists on the inclusion of feticide in the termination process (RCOG 1996 and 2001). This guideline provides a gestational threshold relating to the use of feticide in TOP. We have argued elsewhere (Graham, Robson and Rankin 2008) that while this guideline is sometimes interpreted as the equivalent of a legal requirement the guideline operates in a manner that allows a small amount of professional discretion in determining when a feticide is considered essential. Our findings suggest that, although the guideline on feticide is an important boundary in the decision-making processes that lead to a late TOPFA, it is not necessarily seen as an impassable barrier. We asked the consultant participants to indicate whether they would see late TOPFA as a legitimate option at 26 weeks gestation, with reference to several different types of foetal anomaly. Later in the questionnaire, we returned to these same foetal anomalies and asked if they would *consider* providing TOPFA without feticide at three different gestational points (21, 23 and 25 weeks). The responses for two of the conditions are presented here, one as an example of a 'lethal' foetal anomaly (Edwards Syndrome) and one that is considered 'non-lethal' (Isolated Down's Syndrome).[2]

Table 16.3 Diversity of views about clinical practice in provision of feticide

	Proportion of respondents indicating support for the legitimacy of an offer of TOP at 26 wks	Proportion of 'TOP supportive @26 wks' respondents who went on to indicate support for considering TOP without feticide (excludes indecipherable responses)		
		@21 wks (i.e. just below RCOG feticide guideline threshold)	*@23 wks (i.e. just above RCOG feticide guideline threshold)*	*@25 wks (i.e. above the 24wk viability threshold)*
Condition				
Edwards Syndrome (a 'lethal' anomaly)	60/62 (97%)	26/56 (46%)	21/56 (42%)	17/56 (30%)
Isolated Down's Syndrome (a 'non-lethal' anomaly)	35/61 (57%)	25/32 (71%)	2/32 (6%)	0

2 It should be noted that the use of the term 'lethal' in association with anomalies such as Edwards Syndrome has received some criticism as part of a wider debate on whether the term is technically accurate. For example, Koogler et al. (2003) have highlighted that the use of the term 'lethal' may be problematic as survival rates increase. In contrast, Dommergues et al. (2010: 532) continue to use the term 'lethal', but qualify this with a threshold risk of infant or perinatal death.

From these results, it is clear that there is diversity in terms of why consultants are prepared to provide termination for foetal anomaly, with more consensus for the lethal anomaly than for the non-lethal anomaly. But even within that consensus of offering TOPFA for Edwards Syndrome, there is still considerable variation on whether clinicians would consider providing termination of pregnancy without a feticide. We also provided space for participants to tell us about the factors that would be important to a decision to act 'beyond' the guideline. The responses indicated that many of the consultants kept close to the guideline, but would sometimes consider providing feticide below the standard gestational threshold, and would sometimes consider providing termination of pregnancy without feticide above the standard gestational threshold. The issues raised by these diversions from the guideline are different, but consultants similarly tended to provide a rationale relating to clinical issues (e.g. the weight of the baby, the lethality of the condition) for these diversions.

Dealing with Diversity in Reproductive Loss

The concept of reproductive loss is valuable in terms of bringing together experiences and accounts of bereavement across the spectrum of reproductive health. But this concept encompasses insight into a set of experiences which are experienced and understood by those most closely involved in diverse ways. The examples demonstrate the challenge in using concepts that can encompass the spectrum of understandings in any one particular group (for example, health professionals or bereaved parents, within or across a particular speciality). There is a sense of instability to the key concepts of the reproductive loss narrative, perhaps exemplified best by the ongoing debates about the correct term to refer to the foetus/baby (see Blizzard 2007), or futile attempts to rank severity of bereavement between different categories of loss (e.g. miscarriage versus stillbirth) or foetus/baby (for example, in terms of gestation). For researchers, the field of reproductive loss is important because our data demonstrate the need to use experiences to inform the development of health care that has sufficient flexibility to accommodate difference and individuality within a broader context of consistently good quality care. To make sense of diversity in these settings, and the corresponding need for an appropriate level of professional discretion, the methodological framework of investigation needs to be able to encompass multiple and competing meanings of key issues such as the status of the foetus/baby, and the ways in which pregnant women construct their identities. At the least, this requires a broadly interpretative approach, and we have found that there is value in combining this more established type of qualitative health research approach with an explicitly post-structuralist layer (drawing on Young's description of 'reading against the grain' 1990: 163) to tease out and explore areas of competing meanings.

One area where the value of 'reading against the grain' is evident is in considering how clinical guidelines have a peculiar role in decision making about care pathways and care options. On the one hand, they are used to improve consistency of standards and effectiveness in healthcare delivery across different providers, whether that is at the level of institution, region or something else. But, although guidelines may be important in determining the reasonableness of a clinical decision or intervention, such guidelines do not function as law; they are a marker that aids the interpretation of others, who may or may not be clinicians, about the legitimacy of a course of action. For example, there are mixed views about the ways in which guidelines inform clinical negligence cases (see Jackson 2010: 122-124) but centre around the capacity for guidelines to *become* definitive suggesting that – for now at least – they are not. Recent debates about the content of particular guidelines that relate to reproductive loss (such as the debate on the extent to which parents should be offered the opportunity (rather than encouraged to) to hold their baby after death) and the role of guidelines in informing practice (for example how feticide guidelines are interpreted) reflect the tensions evident in the use of guidelines to inform practice. A key aspect of debates around legitimate practice is the issue of equality. In part, the debates about guidelines in the field of reproductive loss seem to reflect a more established debate in social theory around social action that balances the key components of structure and agency. First, social structures are recognised in terms of the principle of equality, in the sense that all individuals should be treated equally; for those who belong to a social group that is conventionally associated with suffering discrimination, the principle of similar treatment for all is an important safeguard. However, on the other hand, there is a risk that care provision or decision making can become *too* structured in the field of reproductive loss, as bereaved parents may wish to exercise individual agency, demonstrated in preferences over the detail of how they interpret the characteristics needed for sensitive care. From this perspective, guidelines that are too prescriptive in attempting to bring about consistency may be experienced as 'routine' care that does not adequately accommodate the individual, and personal, aspects of experiencing loss.

There is voluminous literature on the merits of evidence based practice and the need for consistency of good quality care; but there is room for improvement in developing the 'evidence base' on how evidence-based medicine could and should be balanced with workable concepts of clinical and personal discretion in responding to complex clinical events such as reproductive loss (an issue that is hardly new, see for example Stradling and Davies 1997). A key aspect of developing an evidence base to inform clinical practices is to develop frameworks of analysis that do more than describe diversity; but which, at the same time, guard against theorising reproductive loss in ways that allow dominant conceptualisations of the loss experience to be used to inform 'best' practice – such developments have the potential to result in unwarranted restriction of professionals' ability to respond to individual cases. In dealing with the diversity evident in experiences of reproductive loss, one of the key challenges for researchers and practitioners alike is to balance adequately the principles of evidence-based health care and equal access to care, with the principle of tolerating differences in how people conceptualise their experiences of reproductive loss.

References

Ajetunmobi, O. 2002. *Making Sense of Critical Appraisal.* London: Hodder Arnold.

ARC. [Online]. Available at: http://www.arc-uk.org/ [accessed: 25 November 2011].

Association of Early Pregnancy Units. 2007. *Guidelines*. AEPU. [Online]. Available at: http://www.earlypregnancy.org.uk/default.asp [accessed: 25 November 2011].

BLISS. [Online] Available at: http://www.bliss.org.uk/ [accessed 1 October 2011].

Blizzard, D. 2007. *Looking Within: A sociocultural examination of fetoscopy.* Cambridge: MA and London: MIT press.

Bolton, S. 2005. Women's work, dirty work: the gynaecology nurse as 'other'. *Gender, Work, Organisation*, 12, 169-186.

Cameron, M., Penney, G., Maclennan, G., McLeer, S. and Walker, A. 2007. Impact on maternity professionals of novel approaches to clinical audit feedback. *Evaluation and the Health Professions*, 30, 75-95.

Chiapetta-Swanson, C. 2005. Dignity and dirty work: nurses' experiences in managing genetic termination for foetal anomaly. *Qualitative Sociology*, 28(1), 93-115.

CMACE. (Centre for Maternal and Child Health Enquiries) 2011. London: CMACE.

Department of Health (DH). [Online]. Available at http://www.dh.gov.uk/en/Publicationsandstatistics/Statistics/StatisticalWorkAreas/Statisticalpublichealth/index.htm [accessed: 25 November 2011].

2003. *Statistical Bulletin: Abortion statistics, England and Wales, 2002.*

2004. *Statistical Bulletin: Abortion statistics, England and Wales, 2003.*

2005. *Statistical Bulletin: Abortion statistics, England and Wales, 2004.*

2006. *Statistical Bulletin: Abortion statistics, England and Wales, 2005.*

2007. *Statistical Bulletin: Abortion statistics, England and Wales, 2006.*

2008. *Statistical Bulletin: Abortion statistics, England and Wales, 2007.*

2009. *Statistical Bulletin: Abortion statistics, England and Wales, 2008.*

2010. *Statistical Bulletin: Abortion statistics, England and Wales, 2009.*

2011. *Statistical Bulletin: Abortion statistics, England and Wales, 2010.*

Dommergues, M., Mandelbrot, L., Mahieu-Caputo, D., Boudjema, N., Durand-Zaleski, I. And the ICI Group-Club de Médecine foetale. 2010. Termination of pregnancy following prenatal diagnosis in France: how severe are the fetal anomalies? *Prenatal Diagnosis*, 30, 531-39.

Earle, S., Komaromy, C., Foley, P. and Lloyd, C.E. 2007. Understanding reproductive loss. Part I: Social dimensions. *The Practising Midwife*, 10(6), 28-34.

Graham, R., Mason, K., Rankin, J. and Robson, S. 2009. The role of feticide in the context of late termination of pregnancy: a qualitative study of health professionals' and parents' views. *Prenatal Diagnosis*, 27, 622-8.

Graham, R., Robson, S. and Rankin, J. 2008. Understanding feticide: an analytic review. *Social Science and Medicine*, 66, 289-300.

Greenhalgh, T. 2006. *How to Read a Paper: the basics of evidence-based medicine*. 3rd Edition. Malden, MA and Oxford: BMJ Books and Blackwell.

Harden, A. and Ogden, J. 1999. Young women's experiences of arranging and having abortions. *Sociology of Health and Illness*, 21(4), 426-44.

Henley, A. and Schott, J. 2009. After stillbirth – offering choices, creating memories. *British Journal of Midwifery*, 17(12), 798-801.

Hinshaw, K., Fayyad, A. and Munjuluri, P. 2006. *The Management of Early Pregnancy Loss: Green Top Guideline*. London: Royal College of Obstetricians and Gynaecologists.

Hunter, B. 2005. Emotion work and boundary maintenance in hospital-based midwifery. *Midwifery*, 21, 253-66.

Jackson, E. 2010. *Medical Law: texts, cases and materials*. 3rd Edition. Oxford and New York: Oxford University Press.

Koogler, T., Wilfond, B. and Friedman Ross, L. 2003. Lethal language, lethal decisions. *Hastings Center Report*, 33(2), 37-41.

Lee, E. 2003. *Abortion, Motherhood and Mental Health: Medicalizing reproduction in the United States and Great Britain*. New York: Aldine de Gruyter.

Midwifery News. 2010. SANDS, The stillbirth and neonatal death charity, welcomes NICE publication of clarification statement on seeing and holding a stillborn baby. [Online]. Available at: http://www.midirs.org/development/midwiferyweb.nsf/link/317645F5C933BF248025774D003CC36A [accessed: 25 November 2011].

RCOG. 1996. *Termination of Pregnancy for Foetal Abnormality*. [Online]. London: RCOG. Available at: http://www.rcog.org.uk/termination-pregnancy-foetal-abnormality-england-scotland-and-wales [accessed: 25 November 2011].

RCOG. 2001. *Further issues relating to late abortion, foetal viability and registration of births and deaths*. [Online]. London: RCOG. Available at: http://www.rcog.org.uk/womens-health/clinical-guidance/further-issues-relating-late-abortion-fetal-viability-and-registration [accessed: 25 November 2011].

Rubington, E. and Weinburg, M. 1989. *The Study of Social Problems: six perspectives* 4th Edition. New York and Oxford: Oxford University Press.

Sands. [Online]. Available at: http://uk-sands.org/ [accessed: 25 November 2011].

Schott, J. and Henley, A. 2008. Seeing and holding a stillborn baby. *British Journal of Midwifery*, 16(9), 593.

Silverman, D. 2006. *Interpreting Qualitative Data*. 3rd Edition. London: Sage.

Simmons, R., Singh, G., Maconochie, N., Doyle, P. and Green, J. 2006. Experience of miscarriage in the UK: qualitative findings from the National Women's Health Study. *Social Science and Medicine*, 63, 1934-46.

Statham, H., Solomou, W. and Green, J. 2006. Late termination of pregnancy: Law, policy and decision making in four English foetal medicine units. *British Journal of Obstetrics and Gynaecology*, 113(12), 1402-1411.

Stradling, J. and Davies, R. 1997. The unacceptable face of evidence-based medicine (guest editorial). *Journal of Evaluation in Clinical Practice*, 3(2), 99-103.

Sur, S. and Raine-Fenning, N. 2009. The management of miscarriage. *Best Practice and Research Clinical Obstetrics and Gynaecology*, 23(4), 479-91.

Walter, T. 2003. Historical and cultural variants on the good death. *British Medical Journal*, 327, 218-20.

Wilcox, A., Weinburg, C., O'Connor, J., Baird, D., Schlatterer, J., Canfield, R. et al. 1988. Incidence of early loss of pregnancy. *New England Medical Journal*, 319(4), 189-94.

Young, A. 1990. *Femininity in Dissent*. London: Routledge.

Index

Reference to the figure is given in italic and tables are in bold.